FRONTRUNNERS' INTERNAL MEDICINE Q&A REVIEW: SELF-ASSESSMENT & BOARD REVIEW

BRADLEY MITTMAN, M.D.

THIRD EDITION

FRONTRUNNERS PUBLISHING/FBRI
23511 Aliso Creek Rd. Suite 93
Aliso Viejo, CA 92656

PREFACE

Welcome to FRONTRUNNERS INTERNAL MEDICINE Q&A REVIEW, designed to prepare you for the **MEDICINE BOARDS** as well as the medicine and subspecialty components of the **USMLE STEPS** 2 & 3. Students who are preparing for the USMLE and are thinking about a residency in medicine as well as current medicine residents will ALSO be *way ahead* of the game when it comes time to sit for their **medicine boards** (yes, there's actually one more exam after step 3 (!) and it's the all-important one that makes you "board-certified"). This book is an excellent **companion** to the Frontrunners Internal Medicine Board Review Syllabus, which remains the syllabus for the Frontrunners Board Review courses that are held throughout the year. While designed with the boards in mind, these resources are nonetheless outstanding study aids for **medical students, residents, and practicing internists** who simply want *the best no-nonsense and most realistic Q&A review of internal medicine in all of its subspecialties.* And for those who are simply looking to expand their fund of knowledge in medicine, this back is without compare, and is ideal for health care professionals at all levels, including nursing practitioners and physician assistants. If you're a mnemonics fan (and who isn't?) and you're prepping for the boards, then you'll *definitely* want to check out **TURBO MNEMONICS FOR THE BOARDS:** Memory Aids to Commonly Asked **CLINICAL** Material You GOTTA Know for the USMLE & Medicine Boards. It features 100s of mnemonics that, we promise, will make your life a whole lot easier. Over the years, we've been blessed with hundreds of questions and answers material that have been voluntarily submitted by physicians who have gone on to pass their boards, in their effort to help those "soldiers left behind"! We have therefore pooled for you from our database all the questions amassed to date, with the answers and explanations as appropriate. This ongoing feedback not only continues to make our board review course progressively stronger but has helped physicians pass this at-times seemingly impossible hurdle called the boards.

This critical board review resource is chock-full of ***over 1,200*** internal medicine board-oriented ***questions*** for you to review before you physically sit for your exam, because, just as important as knowing your "stuff" is being psychologically prepared. Equally important, this review will prepare you for the "all *except* ", "next best step", and multiple choice-type questions and answers *that are now customary* on the exams. While this Q&A review is an excellent companion to the Frontrunners syllabus, the two need not be used together. These Frontrunners "warm-up exercises" will prepare you well for the essential material that you can expect to find on the Internal medicine boards. We've made every effort to make this as simple a resource as possible, with its thorough INDEX section, fully understanding that your time, by virtue of being a student, resident, or practicing internist (if nothing else!), is limited. In our efforts, therefore, to incorporate as much of this material as possible into your review in as succinct a manner as possible, you will find explanations to questions where explanations are due, and not simply to "just fill space". The explanations will not serve to simply reiterate the entire core of the syllabus, but rather to shed light as needed. Except for the length of the questions, which we've intentionally abbreviated in order for you *maximize* your content exposure in *as little time* as possible, you'll see that the *substance* of the material here intimately approximates that which you will see on your exam and will serve as the ideal litmus test of your readiness.

Having said all this, we also realize that there are individuals who have, over the years, grown weary of tedious self-study and who want to take advantage of a sit-down, "feed-me" style of board review, with all the same core material, slides, cases, and more, even if the syllabus can come to them. For this reason we continue to offer our formal / sit-down board review courses throughout the year. These are Saturday & Sunday **WEEKEND MARATHON REVIEWS**, offered each year in March/April, early August, and October—ideal for most physicians who can only spare a weekend; that weekend, however, covers 18 hours of highly intensive review and is not for the faint of heart. For upcoming dates/registration for any of these WEEKEND MARATHON REVIEWS, or to order 1) **TURBO MNEMONICS FOR THE BOARDS**, featuring > 400 anagrams and other mnemonics to markedly improve the efficiency of your board review studying; or 2) the **Q&A REVIEW, featuring > 1200 Q&A**, see the "*Quick Order Form*" at the very end of this book or just call **866-MDBOARDs** to order or inquire.

With greatest wishes for you,

Bradley D. Mittman, MD

Bradley D. Mittman, MD
FRONTRUNNERS BOARD REVIEW, INC.

• NOTICE •

This book is designed as a study aid for residents and physicians who are preparing to take their MEDICINE BOARDS or the medicine and subspecialty components of the USMLE steps 2 & 3. It is also ideal for medical students and residents who are aiming to increase their fund of knowledge in internal medicine. This book is not intended to serve as a complete or standard textbook of internal medicine nor any subspecialties, but rather as a resource to assist the physician in his or her review specifically for the exam. It is in no way intended to be used as the sole reference for one's study or practice of internal medicine nor any subspecialties. Neither the author nor the publisher can be held accountable for any student's or students' individual board scores, as it is expected that all students will invest significant time in personal review of this and other materials such as general textbooks of medicine.

Medicine is an ever-changing science. As new research and clinical experience broaden our knowledge, changes in the treatment and drug therapy are required The author and publisher of this work have checked with sources believed to be reliable in their efforts to provide information that is complete and generally in accord with the standards accepted at the time of publication. However, in view of the possibility of human error or changes in medical sciences, neither the author nor the publisher nor any other party who has been involved in the preparation or publication of this work warrants that the information contained herein is in every respect accurate or complete, and they are not responsible for any errors or omissions or for the results obtained from use of such information. Readers are encouraged to confirm the information contained herein with other sources. This is particularly true insofar as drug selection and dosage are concerned. The reader is urged to check the package insert for each drug for any change in indications or contraindications, dosage, warnings, precautions, or drug-drug interactions.

Dedication

To you Dad, my strongest advocate,
who worked so hard to give me every
opportunity to excel in life, showed
incredible patience, believed in me
thoroughly, and ultimately, taught me
all the great lessons.
I miss you every day.

TABLE OF CONTENTS

HEMATOLOGY QUESTIONS

1. All of the following are clinical features of TTP (Thrombotic Thrombocytopenic Purpura) *except*:
   a) Fever
   b) Renal damage
   c) Microangiopathic hemolytic anemia
   d) Elevated liver enzymes
   e) Thrombocytopenia

2. Which of the following statements is *not* true regarding the presence of schistocytes on peripheral blood smear:
   a) Schistocytes may be seen all of the following diseases: acute renal failure, DIC, hemolytic uremic syndrome, HELLP syndrome, SLE, and PAN.
   b) Schistocytes appear as RBC fragments on the peripheral blood smear.
   c) Pathologically, schistocytes are the result of microangiopathic hemolytic anemia.
   d) Schistocytes in the blood manifest as a Coombs positive anemia.

3. All of the following are true statements regarding the Philadelphia chromosome *except*:
   a) The Philadelphia chromosome is the hallmark of CML.
   b) The Philadelphia chromosome is a 9/22 translocation.
   c) The Philadelphia chromosome results in the formation of a chimeric bcr-abl gene resulting in aggressive differentiation.
   d) The Philadelphia chromosome confers a good prognosis in CML.
   e) The Philadelphia chromosome bears a poor prognosis in AML.

4. Find the statement that is *least* likely to be true regarding the "1 to 1 dilution test":
   a) It is ordered when either the PT or the PTT is elevated.
   b) It is checked in order to ascertain the presence of factor deficiencies versus a factor inhibitor.
   c) When it corrects, you have to look for a factor inhibitor. When it does not correct, it implies the presence of a factor deficiency.
   d) Factor VIII inhibitor, lupus anticoagulant, and antiphospholipid antibody are all factor inhibitors.

5. Choose the incorrect statement from among the following answers regarding delayed transfusion reactions:
   a) It is caused by antibody in the recipient vs. foreign-donor serum proteins.
   b) The Coombs test is positive.
   c) Approximately 1/3rd of patients are asymptomatic. The rest can show any combination of scleral icterus, jaundice, malaise, fatigue, ↑LDH, fever, chills, and anemia.
   d) The reaction does not appear immediately but may take as long as 8 hours to appear after the reaction.

6. Regarding H.A.T.T. (Heparin Associated Thrombocytopenia with Thrombosis), which of the following is *not* a true statement:
   a) Heparin may enhance platelet aggregation causing low platelet count and thrombosis.
   b) Pathologically, the cause is heparin-specific IgG reacting vs. the heparin-platelet complex
   c) The median time for H.A.T.T. to develop after initiating heparin is approximately 2 days.
   d) Because of H.A.T.T., a CBC should be checked each day that a patient is on heparin. The treatment is to stop the heparin once recognized.

7. All of the following regarding PNH (Paroxysmal Nocturnal Hemoglobinuria) are true *except*:
   a) PNH is a chronic disease resulting from an, as yet, unknown defect in the RBC.
   b) Hemolysis is intravascular, yielding Hgbemia and Hgburia.
   c) Non-Hodgkin's lymphoma may develop in 5-10% of patients with PNH.
   d) 50% of deaths due to PNH are associated with venous thromboembolism, including hepatic vein thrombosis.
   e) Aplastic anemia can be the initial hematologic manifestation of this disease. PNH can also develop months to years after the diagnosis of aplastic anemia. The mechanisms whereby PNH induces aplastic anemia are unknown.

8. Which of the following statements is *least* likely to be true regarding Vitamin B12 deficiency?
   a) Homocysteine and MMA (methylmalonic acid) are the first laboratory abnormalities to be seen, even before a drop in the serum vit B12.
   b) Hypersegmented neutrophils typically appear following the elevation in MCV.
   c) Patients symptomatic from vit B12 deficiency need not have abnormal MCV or hematocrit.
   d) There is an increased risk of malignancy in patients with pernicious anemia.
   e) Pernicious anemia may be screened for by checking anti-intrinsic factor (IF) antibodies in the serum.

9. All of the following statements regarding Hemolytic uremic syndrome (HUS) are true *except*:
   a) The clinical findings are often difficult to differentiate from TTP.
   b) Clinically, one looks for fever, thrombocytopenia, and renal involvement..
   c) Management in adults is very similar to that of TTP.
   d) Hemorrhagic colitis may be seen in association with E. Coli 0157-H7, which may be contracted via ingestion of tainted beef or cow products.

10. Which of the following statements regarding sickle cell trait is inaccurate?

a) Patients with sickle cell trait (approximately 8% of blacks) may present with painless hematuria.
b) There is an increased risk of infections in patients who carry the sickle cell trait.
c) Patients with sickle cell *trait* have difficulty concentrating their urine (hypo/isosthenuria).
d) There is no increase in mortality among individuals with sickle cell trait.

11. All of the following statements are true regarding the crises in sickle cell anemia except:

a) Vasoocclusive crisis is the most frequent crisis.
b) Aplastic crisis is usually 2° to bone marrow suppression from a viral infection.
c) Hemolytic crisis is usually 2° to infection or drugs and may be reflected in the labs by an ↑ reticulocyte count, ↑indirect bilirubin, and jaundice.
d) Sequestration crisis refers to the massive pooling of RBCs in the spleen , which generally precedes the autosplenectomy stage of sequestration crisis.

12. A 67 year old female presents to your office with complaints of only weakness and fatigue and "swollen glands" in her neck. Examination reveals right cervical lymphadenopathy and a palpable spleen tip. Her WBC count is 14, 000 and hemoglobin is 9.8 g/dl. The rest of the CBC is completely normal. Cervical lymph node biopsy reveals chronic lymphocytic leukemia. Given all of the above information, you suspect her Rai stage *most likely* to be:

a) Rai stage 0
b) Rai stage I
c) Rai stage II
d) Rai stage III
e) Rai stage IV

13. For the patient listed above in question #12, what is the next best step in managing the CLL at this stage?
a) Tell the patient that the median survival time is 5 years from the onset of treatment and that treatment at this stage would be futile.
b) Let her know that at her early stage, chemotherapy is not warranted since her platelet count is still normal.
c) Explain that her anemia is part of her CLL and is usually very responsive to iron supplementation and gamma globulin treatment.
d) Refer her to an oncologist for treatment with chlorambucil ± prednisone.

14. All of the following are true regarding hairy cell leukemia except:
    a) Peripheral blood smears often show a "fried egg" appearance to cells that stain with tartrate-resistant acid phosphatase.
    b) Bone marrow aspirations often reveal a hypercellular marrow with an abundance of immature white cell precursors.
    c) The leukemia is primarily a B cell disease.
    d) Patients tend to manifest with cytopenias and splenomegaly.
    e) Neutropenias tend to predispose these patients to atypical bacterial infections like legionella, toxoplasmosis, and nocardia.

15. All of the following are true regarding Hodgkin's disease except:
    a) 20-50% of patients will show EBV incorporated into their genome.
    b) Staging is based on sites of involvement.
    c) The treatment for bulky stage II disease is radiation.
    d) A patient with stage IV disease who receives chemotherapy may secondarily develop acute myelogenous leukemia.

16. Each of the following is considered a key independent prognosticator for overall survival in Non-Hodgkin's Lymphoma except:
    a) Age (under or over 40)
    b) Stage (I or II vs. III or IV)
    c) LDH (normal or elevated)
    d) Performance status of the patient (0 or 1 vs. 2 to 4)
    e) Extranodal involvement (no more than 1 site vs. >1 site)

17. All of the following are true regarding Monoclonal Gammopathies of Uncertain Significance (MGUS) except:
    a) One of the key elements differentiating MGUS from multiple myeloma is the quantity of plasma cells found in the bone marrow (≥20% in MM; <20% in MGUS).
    b) MGUS is much more common than myeloma.
    c) Patients with MGUS usually have no urinary Bence Jones protein, no anemia, no renal failure, no hypercalcemia, and no lytic bone lesions.
    d) With long-term follow-up, about 25 percent of patients with MGUS go on to develop myeloma.

18. All of the following are true regarding Multiple Myeloma except:
    a) M protein is usually > 3g/dl, as opposed to <3g/dl in MGUS.
    b) Weakness and fatigue are the most frequent symptoms.
    c) Xrays typically reveal a lytic appearance.
    d) There is an increased risk of pneumococcal infection.
    e) Because multiple myeloma is not curable, treatment should be delayed until evidence of progression is seen.

19. All of the following are true regarding the myeloproliferative disorders except:
    a) They include primary thrombocytosis, polycythemia vera, myelofibrosis, and chronic myelocytic leukemia.
    b) All of them can lead to AML.
    c) The LAP scores in all of these are increased except in P. Vera.
    d) Each involves the clonal expansion of a multipotent hematopoietic progenitor cell with the overproduction of one or more of the formed elements of the blood.

20. All of the following are true regarding Chronic Myelogenous Leukemia except:
    a) The Philadelphia chromosome (t 5,22) is the hallmark of the disease.
    b) This translocation results in premature termination of granulocyte maturation and also results in blast crisis.
    c) Chronic phase is characterized by < 10% blasts in blood and bone marrow.
    d) The disease is characterized by the inevitable transition from a chronic phase to an accelerated phase and on to blast crisis.
    e) Blast crisis is defined as progression to acute leukemia with blood or marrow blasts ≥30%.

21. In the initial treatment of CML, hydroxyurea and α interferon are generally preferred over busulfan because of all of the following potential side effects of busulfan except:
    a) Veno-occlusive disease
    b) Pulmonary, endocardial, and marrow fibrosis
    c) Cushing's-like syndrome
    d) Myelosuppression

22. All of the following are true for Polycythemia Vera except:
    a) There is an increase in RBC mass.
    b) Patients often manifest with a post bathing pruritis.
    c) The erythopoetin level is usually increased.
    d) Splenomegaly is a key diagnostic criteria.
    e) The B12 level is usually increased.

23. In von Willebrand's Disease, all of the following are true statements except:
    a) It is the most common inherited bleeding disorder.
    b) It manifests with a prolonged bleeding time and an elevated PTT.
    c) vWF (von Willebrand factor) is decreased, accounting for the prolonged bleeding time.
    d) dDAVP (desmopressin) is the treatment of choice for minor bleeding.

24. All of the following are true for DIC except:
    a) It is characterized by microvascular clotting secondary to thrombin deposition.
    b) There is an increased PT and PTT secondary to decreased production of clotting factors.
    c) Fibrinogen levels are typically decreased.
    d) DIC is a classic complication of AML, M3.

25. All of the following are true statements relating to Factor XIII deficiency except:
    a) Patients usually bleed in the neonatal period from their umbilical stump or circumcision.
    b) All routine clotting tests are normal except for an elevated PTT.
    c) One should suspect it in cases of delayed post-op bleeding (e.g. after a patient returns home at night following an apparently uncomplicated dental procedure)
    d) If you suspect this disease, a urease clot solubility test may be performed.

26. All of the following are true for Factor V Deficiency except:
    a) It accounts for as many as 5% of "idiopathic" venous thrombosis.
    b) It is also known as the Leiden deficiency.
    c) It is also called hereditary activated protein C resistance (aPC resistance).
    d) It is present in 2-5% of the general population and should be ruled out in patients with DVT who are either pregnant or on oral contraceptives.

Factors 5, 8, and 9 levels have been used to distinguish between the acquired factor deficiencies of liver disease, DIC, and vitamin K deficiency. For questions #27-29, match the acquired factor deficiency to "A", "B", or "C".

	"A"	"B"	"C"
Factor V	↓	↓	normal
Factor VIII	normal	↓	normal
Factor IX	↓	↓	↓

27.DIC

28.Liver disease

29.Vitamin K deficiency

30. All of the following decrease the warfarin level when used concomitantly except:
    a) Sulfonamides
    b) Barbiturates
    c) Carbamazepine
    d) Rifampin

DVT prophylaxis is important and varies by patient situation. For questions #31-34, match each of the following recommendations to the correct patient population.

A. Early ambulation
B. Low-dose unfractionated heparin (LDUH) or low molecular-weight heparin (LMWH), combined with intermittent pneumatic compression (IPC)
C. LMWH, started 12-24h postop; or warfarin, started before or immediately after surgery or adjusted-dose heparin, started preoperatively
D. LDUH or LMWH

31. General medical patients with clinical risk factors for DVT, particularly those with CHF or chest infections.
32. Low-risk general surgery patients.
33. Patients undergoing total hip replacement.
34. Very-high-risk general surgery patients with multiple risk factors.

35. In aplastic anemia all of the following are true statements except:
    a) The bone marrow is typically hypocellular.
    b) Mortality is 80% at 2 years unless the patient receives either bone marrow transplant or ATG (antithymocyte globulin).
    c) It can be associated with hepatitis B or C.
    d) If transfusions are needed, attempt to select related donors whenever possible.

36. All of the following are true regarding ITP (Idiopathic Thrombocytopenic Purpura) except:
    a) Drugs commonly implicated include procainamide, quinine, quinidine, heparin, gold, sulfonamides, and rifampin.
    b) High dose gamma globulin works by decreasing the number of phagocytic cell Fc receptors..
    c) The mainstay of treatment is steroids.
    d) Splenectomy may be done to remove the predominant site of antibody production and platelet destruction.

37. All of the following are true statements in hemochromatosis except:
    a) The best screening modality is serum transferrin saturation.
    b) Arthropathy and hypogonadism are *both* among the irreversible complications of the disease.
    c) The pathogenesis is felt to be related to ferritin, the transferrin receptor, and the iron regulatory protein involved in the coordinated regulation of ferritin and the transferrin receptor.
    d) Hemochromatosis is one of the most common autosomal recessive disorders.
    e) In the liver of patients with hemochromatosis, parenchymal iron is in the form of ferritin and hemosiderin.

38. All of the following may cause hemolysis in G6PD-deficient individuals except:
    a) Primaquine
    b) Dapsone
    c) Sulfamethoxazole
    d) Doxorubicin
    e) Cephalosporins

39. Each of the following clotting factors may be found in the Final Common Pathway except:
    a) Factor VII
    b) Factor X
    c) Factor II
    d) Factor V

For the next set of questions, match each hypochromic anemia with the correct set of indices.

	Serum Fe	**TIBC**	**Serum Ferritin**	**Bone Marrow Fe**
A.	↓	↑	↓	↓
B.	↓	↓	Normal	Normal
C.	Normal	Normal	Normal	Normal
D.	↑	Normal	↑	↑

40. α or β thalassemia trait
41. Chronic inflammation or malignancy
42. Iron deficiency
43. Sideroblastic anemia

44. All of the following are examples of hematologic diseases that can cause cerebral infarction except:
    a) Leukemia
    b) Essential thrombocythemia
    c) TTP
    d) Multiple myeloma

1. All of the following are classic prognosticators when talking about tumor features associated with breast carcinoma except:
   a) High mitotic activity (high S phase)
   b) Large tumor (>1.5cm)
   c) Undifferentiated/poorly differentiated histopathology
   d) Tumor adherent to the skin/chest wall/pectoralis muscle
   e) Her2neu receptor status

2. Among all the prognosticators studied in breast carcinoma, in general, which of the following is the most reliable:
   a) Size of the primary tumor
   b) Clinical symptomatology
   c) Positive axillary lymph nodes
   d) Histology (ductal vs. lobular)
   e) ER/PR receptor status

3. A patient who reports a 2 week history of blood in his stool undergoes a full colonoscopy by his gastroenterologist that reveals a 2.5 cm sessile mass at the splenic flexure. Biopsy reveals colorectal carcinoma that has extended through the serosa. Which of the following would you recommend for him:

   a) Surgery plus chemotherapy
   b) Surgery alone
   c) Surgery plus radiation
   d) Endoscopic exfulguration and follow-up in 3 months
   e) Chemotherapy alone

4. Lung carcinoma is renown for its array of paraneoplastic phenomena. All of the following paraneoplastic features are known to be associated with small cell lung carcinoma except:
   a) Carcinoid syndrome
   b) Cushing's syndrome
   c) SIADH
   d) Eaton-Lambert syndrome
   e) Hypercalcemia

5. All of the following are true regarding the staging and treatment of small and non-small cell lung carcinoma except:
   a) The reason for the small cell vs. non-small cell nomenclature has to do with the differences in staging and management.
   b) Stage II non-small cell lung ca has positive hilar lymph nodes and is considered resectable.
   c) Stage IIIB non-small cell lung ca is an important stage because the cancer has now spread to the contralateral side and is no longer deemed operable.
   d) Limited disease small cell lung carcinoma responds well to a combination of surgery and chemo in most cases.

6. Important criteria in determining operability in lung cancer patients include all of the following except:

   a) Lung lesion > 2cm from the carina
   b) For preoperative FEV1<3L or DL_{CO} < 60%, a quantitative V/Q scan should be done to assess the expected post-op FEV1, which must be >2L.
   c) Noninvolvement of major vessels
   d) Resting pCO_2 >50

7. In discussing the staging of Hodgkin's Lymphoma, all of the following are true except:
   a) Stage II disease involves ≥ 2 lymph node sets on one side of the diaphragm.
   b) Stages I-IIIA1 respond to radiation therapy alone.
   c) Stage IIIA2 requires chemotherapy.
   d) Radiation therapy alone is a reasonable option for bulky Stage II disease.
   e) It is important to do a laparotomy on all "apparent" stage I and II disease.

8. Those who survive the initial chemotherapy of Hodgkin's Disease may secondarily develop all of the following except:
   a) AML
   b) Diffuse, aggressive lymphomas
   c) Solid tumors
   d) Leiomyosarcomas

9. Low grade Non-Hodgkin's Lymphoma includes all of the following except:

   a) Diffuse large cell lymphoma
   b) CLL
   c) Multiple Myeloma
   d) Waldenstrom's macroglobulinemia

10. Each of the following statements is true about malignant melanoma except:

    a) Individuals with fair skin, dysplastic nevi, a family history, or repeated and/or blistering sun exposure as a child are at risk
    b) A size cutoff of 4mm in diameter is often used to help distinguish benign pigmented lesions from melanoma and its precursors.
    c) A tumor thickness no greater than 0.76 mm is associated with a high chance of survival.
    d) Moh's surgery in melanoma is considered both diagnostic and therapeutic.

11. Regarding the tumor suppressor genes BRCA 1 and 2, which of the following is incorrect:
    a) Mutations to these genes represent 5-10% of all cases of breast carcinoma.
    b) There is an increased relative risk for development of breast carcinoma among men with the BRCA1 mutation.
    c) Women with BRCA1 mutations are at greater relative risk for development of ovarian carcinoma than women with BRCA2 mutations.
    d) Among the many types of patients for whom genetic testing is indicated, one indication is a patient with early onset (<50yo) breast carcinoma of Ashkenazi descent.

12. Revised criteria for the diagnosis of HNPCC (Hereditary Non-Polyposis Colorectal Cancer) stipulate that at least 3 of the patient's relatives must have an HNPCC-associated cancer. All of the following are additional criteria except:
    a) At least one of the 3 should be a first degree relative of the other 2.
    b) At least 2 successive generations should be affected.
    c) At least 1 relative was diagnosed before age 30.
    d) Tumors should be assessed pathologically.

13. Testicular cancer is the #1 cancer among males age 15-35 years old. All of the following are equally true except:
    a) The biggest risk factor is cryptorchidism.
    b) Even if surgically corrected at an early age, cryptorchidism continues to confer an increased relative risk for testicular ca.
    c) Stage IV testicular carcinoma with distant mets to the mediastinum requires chemotherapy and is incurable.
    d) Nonseminomas secrete both αFP (alpha-fetoprotein) and β-HCG.

14. A 19 yo male presents with a painless mass in his left testes. On examination this is an easily palpable, hard mass. Ultrasound confirms the finding, his αFP is negative but his β-HCG is positive, and an ultrasound-guided biopsy reveals a seminoma. The patient undergoes a radical inguinal orchiectomy with exploration, which, when combined with CT staging of the pelvis, places the patient at a Stage III seminoma with 7 positive peritoneal lymph nodes, some greater than 2 cm. What is the next best step in management of this patient?

    a) Reassure the patient that testicular carcinoma has a high rate of spontaneous resolution even at advanced stages and that aggressive measures are unwarranted.
    b) Radiation therapy alone
    c) Platinum-based chemotherapy alone
    d) Surgical removal of all peritoneal and retroperitoneal lymph nodes, checking αFP and β-HCG every 3-6 months.

15. A 62 yo black female presented to her physician with several months of easy fatigability, anorexia, and a change in her bowel habits. Abdominal exam was essentially unremarkable but a rectal exam revealed guaiac positive stool, grossly heme negative. Her hemoglobin was 9.3 g/dl. Otherwise her labs were unremarkable. Subsequent colonoscopy revealed a 5 cm sessile-based colon carcinoma at the hepatic flexure. Biopsy showed extent of the colon carcinoma through the serosa. Surgical exploration revealed pelvic lymph nodes that were completely free of disease. The most appropriate management in this patient would be:
    a) Surgery followed by chemotherapy
    b) Surgical excision of the mass.
    c) Surgery followed by external beam radiation or brachytherapy
    d) Radiation alone.

16. A 61 yo woman presents to her physician complaining of increasing dyspnea over the past 2 months. Chest X-ray shows left hilar lymphadenopathy. Follow-up CT scan reveals additional left-sided mediastinal lymphadenopathy not involving any major vascular structures and located 2.5 cm from the carina, as well as supraclavicular lymphadenopathy. A biopsy of the supraclavicular node reveals non-small cell lung carcinoma. What is the most appropriate management in this patient?
    a) Surgery alone
    b) Chemotherapy alone
    c) Surgery and radiation
    d) Surgery and chemotherapy

17. A 73 yo male is diagnosed with small cell lung carcinoma stage "limited disease". How are patients with limited disease managed?
    a) Surgery alone
    b) Chemotherapy alone
    c) Chemotherapy and radiation
    d) Surgery plus chemotherapy

18. A 38 yo male presents to your office with complaints of fever, chills, night sweats, and weight loss. His PPD is negative (with positive controls), and blood cultures are negative for endocarditis. When he returns to have his PPD read, his cultures are back and are negative, but he describes a new "lump" in his right neck. Your examination confirms this 2x3cm right supraclavicular mass to be lymphadenopathy, and you suspect lymphoma. Biopsy of that lymph node reveals Hodgkin's Lymphoma. Patient undergoes a staging laparotomy which reveals multiple sets of lymph nodes that biopsy positive above the diaphragm. What is the most appropriate therapeutic recommendation at this time?
    a) External beam radiation followed by chemotherapy
    b) Chemotherapy alone
    c) Surgical excision of all involved lymph nodes
    d) External beam radiation alone

For the following set of questions, match each feature with the correct chronic leukemia, CML or CLL.

A. CML
B. CLL

19. Philadelphia chromosome absent
20. Platelets may be raised, normal, *or* reduced.
21. Serum B12 is raised and B12 binding capacity is increased.
22. Treatment typically includes chlorambucil or cyclophosphamide.

23. A leukemoid reaction is differentiated from CML by all of the following except:

a) Palpable spleen
b) The presence of large numbers of mature neutrophils
c) High LAP score
d) Philadelphia chromosome is absent.

24. All of the following are considered poor prognosticators in multiple myeloma except:

a) BUN > 13 at presentation
b) Hgb > 8g/dl at presentation
c) Serum albumin >3.0
d) Bence-Jones proteinuria >200 mg/dl

25. Each of the following electrolyte abnormalities are commonly seen in the tumor lysis syndrome except:

a) Hyperkalemia
b) Hyperphosphatemia
c) Hypercalcemia
d) Hyperuricemia
e) Raised creatinine and BUN

RHEUMATOLOGY QUESTIONS

1. The differential diagnosis of morning stiffness/pain worse in the AM includes all of the following except:
   a. Polymyalgia rheumatica
   b. Ankylosing Spondylitis
   c. Fibromyalgia
   d. Rheumatoid arthritis
   e. Psoriatic arthritis

2. Charcot's joints (neuropathic arthritides) may be seen in all of the following conditions except:
   a. Syringomyelia
   b. Osteoarthritis
   c. Tabes dorsalis
   d. Diabetes mellitus
   e. Overzealous intraarticular injections of steroids

Questions #3-9 are matching-type questions and address the radiographic signs of Osteoarthritis and Rheumatoid Arthritis. Choose one best answer from the choices below:

A) Osteoarthritis
B) Rheumatoid arthritis
C) Both A and B
D) Neither A nor B

3. Marginal bony erosions
4. Subchondral sclerosis
5. Osteophyte formation
6. Periarticular osteopenia
7. Joint space narrowing
8. Loose bodies
9. Subluxation and gross deformity

10. Each of the following statements about the extraarticular manifestations of Rheumatoid Arthritis are true except:
    a) They are more common among patients with high titres of rheumatoid factor.
    b) Leukocytoclastic vasculitis is an extraarticular manifestation.
    c) RA patients may present with mononeuritis multiplex.
    d) Ocular findings may include episcleritis and uveitis; uveitis is the #1 opthalmic complication.
    e) Caplan's syndrome is a known association.

Questions #11-19 are matching-type questions on DMARD therapy in rheumatoid arthritis and the potential toxicities requiring careful monitoring. Choose one best answer only.

A) Azathioprine
B) Corticosteroids
C) Cyclosporine
D) Etanercept
E) Hydroxycholoroquine
F) Infliximab
G) Methotrexate
H) Minocycline
I) Leflunomide

11. Thrombocytopenia, hepatotoxicity, diarrhea
12. Reactions at the site of the SQ injection, flu-like symptoms
13. Renal insufficiency, anemia, hypertension, hirsutism
14. Flu-like symptoms, autoantibodies, given IV
15. Photosensitivity, skin discoloration, GI upset, drug-induced hepatitis, dizziness
16. Macular damage
17. Myelosuppression, hepatotoxicity, lymphoproliferative disorders
18. Hypertension, cataracts, osteoporosis
19. Myelosuppression, hepatic fibrosis, cirrhosis, pulmonary infiltrates or fibrosis

20. Two clinical entities, Still's disease and Felty's syndrome, are often confused. All of the following statements about the two are correct except:
    a) Usually the WBC is ↑ in Still's disease and ↓ in Felty's syndrome.
    b) High spiking fevers typically accompany Still's disease, whereas fever is not an important part of Felty's syndrome.
    c) Both diseases are seronegative rheumatoid arthritides.
    d) Splenomegaly is commonly seen in both diseases.

21. A number of diseases can give oral and/or genital ulceration. All of the following diseases yield ulcerations that are painful except:
    a) Behcet's disease
    b) Syphilis
    c) Pemphigus
    d) Herpes simplex virus

For questions #22-30, match the appropriate description to the appropriate disease.

A. Reiter's disease
B. Behçet's disease
C. Both
D. Neither

22. HLA association is present
23. Infection plays an important role in pathogenesis
24. Long-term joint disability is frequent.
25. Long-term ocular disability is common.
26. Males are affected more frequently than females.
27. Racial factors important in pathogenesis
28. Spondylitis/sacroiliitis is frequent .
29. The predominant ocular disease is conjunctivitis, as opposed to uveitis.
30. Treatment is NSAIDs.

31. Which of the following is not considered a minor diagnostic criteria for PMR?
    a) Increased alkaline phosphatase or GGTP
    b) Symmetrical proximal muscle weakness
    c) Increased CPK
    d) Normocytic anemia

32. All of the following are true statements regarding PMR or TA (temporal arteritis) except:
    a) 50% of patients with TA have symptoms of PMR.
    b) 10-20% of patients with clinically pure PMR (only symptoms of PMR) will be found to have TA on biopsy.
    c) Half of all PMR patients (with or without concomitant TA symptomatology) will be found to have giant-cell arteritis on TA biopsy.
    d) The appropriate length of segment of TA biopsy, in order to limit the false negatives due to 'skip' lesions, is 1-2 cm.

33. Choose the incorrect statement from among the following ones regarding Temporal Arteritis:
    a) A temporal artery biopsy should be obtained as quickly as possible in the setting of ocular signs and symptoms; however, a biopsy should first be arranged before starting any steroids due to false negative results.
    b) Treatment should begin with prednisone, 15-30 mg per day for approximately 1 month, followed by a gradual tapering to a maintenance dose of 7.5 to 10 mg per day.
    c) Because of the possibility of relapse, therapy should be continued for at least 1 to 2 years.
    d) The ESR can serve as a useful indicator of inflammatory disease activity in monitoring and tapering therapy.

34. Choose the incorrect statement from among the following statements regarding relapsing polychondritis:
    a) Fever, arthralgias, and episcleritis are commonly seen.
    b) 'Ulceration and perforation of the cornea may occur and cause blindness.
    c) A significantly higher frequency of HLA-DR3 has been found in patients with relapsing polychondritis than in normal individuals.
    d) A variety of skin diseases are associated with relapsing polychondritis, including erythema nodosum, erythema multiforme, angioedema/urticaria, and livedo reticularis.

35. Rheumatologic manifestations of sickle cell disease include all of the following except:
    a) Gout
    b) Secondary hemochromatotic arthropathy
    c) Osteomyelitis, most commonly due to pneumococcus, especially in hyposplenic patients
    d) Aseptic necrosis

36. Each of the following is considered a precipitating factor common to gout and pseudogout except:
    a) Trauma
    b) Alcohol
    c) Salicylates
    d) Operation

37. All of the following medical conditions are known to be associated with gout except:
    a) Cholelithiasis
    b) Hypertension
    c) Diabetes mellitus
    d) Atherosclerosis

38. Each of the following medications can be useful in acute attacks of gout except:
    a) Steroids
    b) Probenicid
    c) Allopurinol
    d) Indomethacin

39. Allopurinol has varied toxicities. Among these include all of the following except:
    a) Transaminitis
    b) Renal insufficiency
    c) Fever
    d) Thrombocytosis
    e) Desquamating, erythematous rash

Questions #40-44 are matching-type questions. Match the medication with the appropriate description. Answers may be used once, more than once, or not at all.

A. Colchicine
B. Indomethacin
C. Probenicid
D. Allopurinol

40. Generally speaking, it is the drug of choice if the patient has a history of renal insufficiency or renal stones.
41. May give severe side effects in its PO form only
42. Should be avoided if a patient has a history of kidney stones or a 24h uric acid level > 1000mg
43. Should be avoided in patients with CHF or PUD
44. Simultaneous administration of aspirin or indomethacin should be avoided if possible.

45. All of the following are diseases associated with calcium pyrophosphate disease except:

a) Hyperparathyroidism
b) Hyperphosphatemia
c) Hemochromatosis
d) Hypothyroidism
e) Wilson's disease

46. All of the following are associated with HLA-B27 except:

a) Ankylosing spondylitis
b) Acute anterior uveitis
c) Juvenile rheumatoid arthritis
d) Behçet's disease
e) Psoriatic arthritis

47. All of the following are accurate descriptions of DISH (**D**iffuse **I**diopathic **S**keletal **H**yperostosis) except:

a) DISH is a form of primary osteoarthritis.
b) Flowing ossification is seen along the anterolateral aspects of at least 4 consecutive vertebral bodies.
c) Disk height is preserved which helps to differentiate it from spondylosis.
d) Patients have stiffness and severe limitations in range of motion.

48. Each of the following is considered a radiographic finding in ankylosing spondylitis except:
    a) Sacroiliitis
    b) Lumbar lordosis
    c) Syndesmophytes
    d) Erosions

49. All of the following are clinical signs associated with Reiter's syndrome except:
    a) Spondyloarthropathy
    b) Circinate balanitis
    c) Keratoderma hemorrhagica
    d) Dactylitis

For questions #50-55 match each rheumatic disease with its correct HLA association

A. DR8
B. DR5
C. Dw4/DR4
D. Dw3
E. DR3
F. DR4

50. Juvenile arthritis, pauciarticular

51. Juvenile RA

52. Rheumatoid arthritis

53. Sjögren's syndrome

54. SLE (caucasians)

55. SLE (hydralazine)

56. All of the following are true regarding arthritis associated with inflammatory bowel disease except:
    a) Spondylitis/sacroiliitis, which occur in about 5% of IBD patients, may predate the onset of bowel symptoms and clinically follow bowel disease activity.
    b) The peripheral arthritis tends to occur ≥ 6 months after the onset of bowel disease.
    c) The severity of the peripheral arthritis reflects that of the bowel disease. Colectomy rids it.
    d) Erythema nodosum, uveitis, oral ulcers, and pyoderma occur in association with peripheral arthritis in IBD.

57. All of the following are true regarding HLA-B27 except:
   a) Among HLA-B27 persons in the general population, only 2-10% will develop spondyloarthropathy.
   b) Patients with IBD alone have an increased incidence of HLA-B27 and, therefore, an increased risk of developing spondylitis.
   c) HLA-B27 is neither necessary nor sufficient in diagnosing ankylosing spondylitis
   d) Among patients with IBD *and* ankylosing spondylitis, 75% are HLA-B27 positive.

58. Reactive arthritis is an aseptic arthritis induced by host response to infectious agents rather than a direct result of infection. From among the following GI/GU system infections, choose the one that is *not* associated with reactive arthritis.
   a) Shigella flexneri
   b) Yersinia enterocolytica
   c) Campylobacter jejuni
   d) Ureaplasma urealyticum
   e) Clostridium difficile

59. All of the following are true statements about Lyme disease except:
   a) Bell's palsy is seen in Stage II.
   b) Arthritis may be seen in stage II or Stage III and is not just Stage III.
   c) The arthritis is recurrent, symmetric, and often affects the knees.
   d) The carditis and Bell's palsy are commonly reversible, and prognosis is usually favorable if seen.

60. Concerning the arthritis of Lyme disease, the following statements are true except for:
   a) Those with chronic joint disease have an association with HLA-DR4.
   b) The synovium resembles that of rheumatoid arthritis.
   c) Obliterative endarteritis is a characteristic feature of Lyme arthritis.
   d) Lyme arthritis generally responds poorly to therapy. However, a regimen of oral doxycycline, oral amoxicillin plus probenecid, or parenteral ceftriaxone for a period of 3 to 4 weeks may be tried.

61. Which of the following statements is *not* true regarding HPOA (Hypertrophic Pulmonary Osteoarthropathy)?
   a) The joint appearance and presentation is generally similar to osteoarthritis.
   b) It may be secondary to lung carcinoma or bacterial endocarditis.
   c) Periosteal new bone formation occurs at the end of long bones, yielding tenderness and soft-tissue swelling.
   d) Lowering the legs characteristically improves the pain.

62. All of the following are causes of clubbing except:
    a) Hypothyroidism
    b) Cystic fibrosis
    c) Upper extremity AV fistula
    d) Celiac disease

63. The inflammatory myopathies consist of dermatomyositis, polymyositis, and inclusion body myositis. Which of the following statements concerning these conditions is not true:
    a) All of these commonly give proximal muscle weakness.
    b) Inclusion body myositis commonly gives proximal and distal muscle weakness.
    c) All of these respond favorably to steroids.
    d) Dermatomyositis can give poikiloderma.

For the next set of questions regarding complement levels in renal disease vs. systemic disease, choose one best answer "A", "B", "C", or "D" for each disease.

	Low Serum Complement	**Normal Serum Complement**
Primary Renal Disease	A	C
Systemic Disease	B	D

64. Alport's syndrome
65. Berger's disease (IgA nephropathy)
66. Goodpasture's disease
67. HUS
68. Infective endocarditis
69. Membranoproliferative glomerulonephritis
70. Mixed essential cryoglobulinemia
71. Occult abscess
72. Polyarteritis nodosa
73. Poststreptococcal glomerulonephritis
74. Rapidly progressive glomerulonephritis
75. SLE
76. TTP
77. Wegener's disease

78. All of the following statements are true regarding SLE except:
    a) Signs of proliferation, inflammation, or crescent formation usually require treatment.
    b) Anti-ds DNA is the most specific autoantibody for SLE.
    c) Total serum complement decreases with active disease.
    d) Low CH50 levels usually imply skin or renal involvement.

For questions #79-83 match the fluorescence pattern with the correct rheumatic disorder. Choose the one best answer. Choose the one best answer.

A. Homogeneous/diffuse
B. Rim, peripheral
C. Nucleolar
D. Speckled

79. Acute SLE
80. Chronic SLE
81. Mixed connective tissue disease
82. Polymyositis
83. Scleroderma

For questions # 84-91 match each of the following autoantibodies with its associated rheumatic condition. Choose the one BEST answer, from among the choices given, for its primary clinical importance.

A. Anti-ds DNA
B. Anti-RNP
C. Anti-Ro; anti-La
D. Antihistone protein
E. Anti-Scl
F. Anticentromere
G. Anti-Jo
H. Antiribosomal-P protein

84. CREST syndrome
85. Diffuse Scleroderma
86. Drug-induced SLE
87. Mixed Connective Tissue Disease
88. Sjögren's syndrome
89. Most specific for SLE
90. Dermatomyositis
91. SLE CNS psychosis or depression

92. A 58 yo male is placed on 500mg mg twice a day of Procanbid, an extended release procainamide for his ventricular arrhythmias, by his cardiologist. His arrhythmias have not returned since starting this agent. When he returns to his PCP for a scheduled follow-up exam, the patient has no new complaints, and his exam and review of systems are unremarkable. Except for an ANA of 1:640 and an HDL of 65, his labs are within normal limits. The most appropriate management in this patient is:

    a) Decrease the Procanbid to 250mg twice a day and recheck his ANA in 4 weeks.
    b) Decrease the Procanbid to 250mg twice a day and arrange follow-up with his cardiologist.
    c) Discontinue the Procanbid because of your suspicion of drug-induced lupus.
    d) Continue the medicine at current doses with appropriate follow-up visits with his PCP and cardiologist.

93. All of the following are considered potentially therapeutic in managing Raynaud's disease except:

    a) Biofeedback
    b) Beta-blockers
    c) Nitrates
    d) Calcium channel blockers

94. All of the following are considered potential clinical manifestations of antiphospholipid syndrome except:

    a) Thromboangiitis obliterans
    b) Thrombocytopenia
    c) Recurrent fetal loss
    d) Visceral infarction

95. All of the following diseases may be associated with livedo reticularis except:

    a) SLE
    b) Cryofibrinogenemia
    c) Wegener's syndrome
    d) Cholesterol emboli

In comparing primary vs. secondary Raynaud's it's important to recognize the differentiating features. For questions # 96-100, match each characteristic to the correct disease. Choose either A or B.

A. Primary Raynaud's disease
B. Secondary Raynaud's disease

96. Greater preponderance among females
97. Tends to affect a single digit only, as opposed to all digits
98. Attacks are infrequent
99. Frequently precipitated by emotional stress
100. Livedo reticularis commonly associated

101. Raloxifene and Tamoxifen tend to act in concert when it comes to exerting estrogenic vs. antiestrogenic effects on various organs. From among the following organs, choose the one in which raloxifene and tamoxifen do NOT act in conjunction; that is, one is estrogenic and the other antiestrogenic.

    a) Bone
    b) Breast
    c) Endometrium
    d) CNS

102. A 57 yo obese, white, female smoker presents to you with a wrist fracture following what she felt to be minimal trauma. She describes a history of another fracture 3 years ago to her collar bone after bumping into the door of the subway as she was exiting. Based on her profile, you suspect that she may have osteoporosis and order a bone densitometry, which shows a Standard Deviation of 2.7 below the usual reference. In addition to this study, you should rule out all of the following in the workup of her osteoporosis *except*:

    a) Hypothyroidism
    b) Hyperparathyroidism
    c) Diabetes mellitus
    d) Alcoholism

103. By W.H.O. criteria what is the range of bone mineral density, in Standard Deviations (SD) below the young adult reference mean, for osteopenia?

    a) BMD within 1 SD of the reference
    b) BMD between .5 and 1.5 SD below the reference
    c) BMD between 1.5 and 2.0 below the reference
    d) BMD between 1.0 and 2.5 below the reference

104. All of the following are true regarding osteomalacia except:
   a) The pathology is due to failure of mineralization of the bone.
   b) Calcium is decreased, while phosphorous and alk phos are increased.
   c) 'Pseudofractures' are a classic radiographic sign of osteomalacia.
   d) Vitamin D and calcium are important in treatment.

105. All of the following are true for renal osteodystrophy except:
   a) It is caused by secondary hyperparathyroidism.
   b) It is commonly seen in acute renal failure.
   c) A proximal myopathy not uncommonly coexists with the osteitis fibrosa cystica.
   d) The pathophysiology begins with phosphate retention, hypovitaminosis D, and acidosis.

106. All of the following are typical sites of involvement in Paget's bone disease except:
   a) Tibia
   b) Humerus
   c) Sacrum
   d) Wrists

107. Potential for malignant transformation is greatest for what part of the body in Paget's disease:
   a) Skull
   b) Spine
   c) Femur and humerus
   d) Pelvis and sacrum

108. All of the following are true statements about fibromyalgia except:
   a) Patients' awaken in AM feeling poorly rested due to increased nocturnal awakenings.
   b) Pain must be present for at least 3 months.
   c) Patients are poorly able to localize their pain.
   d) Pain is increased in the mornings.

109. Each of the following is a clinical manifestation of PAN (polyarteritis nodosa) except:
   a) Hypogammaglobulinemia
   b) Retinal hemorrhage
   c) Interstitial pneumonitis
   d) Livedo reticularis

110. All of the following are true statements about cryoglobulinemia except:
   a) Generally, the symptoms of Type I cryoglobulinemia are related to hyperviscosity.
   b) Type II is commonly associated with autoimmune disorders and chronic infections.
   c) The usual presentation for Type II includes palpable purpura and urticaria.
   d) Type III is essentially comprised of monoclonal antibodies.

111. Each of the following is true about Churg-Strauss disease except:
   a) Allergic angiitis and granulomatous vasculitis are the characteristic histopathological features.
   b) The vasculitis is limited to medium-to-small sized veinules.
   c) It is very similar to classic PAN, except that lung involvement is predominant.
   d) Clinically recognizable heart disease occurs in approximately one-third of patients.

112. Each of the following is true for Buerger's disease except:
   a) Thromboangiitis obliterans is the histopathology responsible
   b) The prevalence is higher in Asians and individuals of eastern European descent.
   c) The disease is considered a true classic vasculitis.
   d) This disorder develops most frequently in men under age 40 and classically presents with instep claudication.

113. Sjögren's syndrome may be associated with all of the following clinical manifestations except:
   a) Primary biliary cirrhosis
   b) Intestinal lymphangiectasia
   c) Renal tubular acidosis
   d) Lymphoreticular hyperplasia

GASTROENTEROLOGY QUESTIONS

1. All of the following are true regarding arterial venous malformations (AVMs) except:
   a) There is an increased incidence among patients with polycystic kidney disease.
   b) The incidence of AVMs is greater on the right side of the colon than on the left.
   c) There is an increased incidence in patients on dialysis and patients with end-stage renal disease.
   d) There is an increased incidence of AVMs in aortic stenosis.
   e) Cautery is a form of treatment commonly employed.

2. The differential diagnosis of a flapping tremor includes all of the following except:
   a) Uremia
   b) CO_2 narcosis
   c) Hepatic encephalopathy
   d) Wilson's disease
   e) Progressive supranuclear palsy

3. The sudden increase in ascites in a previously stable cirrhotic can be a worrisome sign and classically can include all of the following causes except:
   a) Hepatoma
   b) Spontaneous bacterial peritonitis
   c) Alcoholic cardiomyopathy
   d) Superinfection with hepatitis D
   e) Hepatic vein thrombosis
   f) Hepatorenal syndrome

4. The classic signs of irritable bowel syndrome include all of the following except:
   a) ↑ frequency of bowel movements with situations involving ↑ stress
   b) An urgent need to defecate that may awaken the patient from sleep
   c) Abdominal pain relieved by the passage of stool
   d) Pencil-thin stools
   e) Chronic or recurrent abdominal distension

5. Regarding Hepatitis B serology, all of the following are true statements except:
   a) If a chronic surface antigen carrier presents with an unexplained exacerbation, a delta agent antibody should be requested.
   b) If a patient with long-standing Hep B presents with a sudden increase in ascites, it is reasonable to check an alpha-fetoprotein.
   c) If a patient with chronic Hep B presents with new or sudden-onset abdominal pain that cannot be accounted for by liver disease per se, polyarteritis nodosa should be ruled out.
   d) For chronic hepatitis B, patients must have transaminitis for at least 3 months.

6. All of the following statements regarding hepatitis C are true except:
   a) All positive EIA results must be confirmed with a supplemental assay such as a RIBA or qualitative RT-PCR.
   b) If a patient has a positive EIA but his PCR is negative, a RIBA should be checked in order to distinguish between resolved infection vs. a false positive EIA.
   c) A single HCV RNA test is sufficient to rule out chronic infection in known HCV-infected patients.
   d) HCV genotyping has a role in guiding treatment regimens. Genotype 1 is the most common in the United States and is associated with lower response rates to current therapy.

For questions #7-10, match the Hepatitis C diagnosis to the appropriate set of data:

	ALT	EIA (ELISA)	RIBA	HCV RNA (RT-PCR)
A)	↑	+	+	+
B)	N	+	+	+
C)	N	+	+	-
D)	N	+	-	-

7. False-positive EIA
8. HCV carrier
9. Resolved infection or intermittent viremia
10. Chronic hepatitis C

11. Of the six hepatitis C genomes we know of to date, which one is not only the most common genotype in the U.S., but is *also* associated with lower response rates to current therapy?
    a) Genotype 3
    b) Genotype 2
    c) Genotype 1
    d) Genotype 5

12. All of the following are true regarding hepatitis D except:
    a) HDV can occur as a superinfection in patients with underlying acute HBV or as a coinfection during chronic HBV infection.
    b) HDV is an RNA virus that is unable to replicate on its own and requires HBV.
    c) In hepatitis B coinfection with hepatitis D, the anti-HepB core IgM is positive.
    d) The major significance of HDV is its ability to increase the severity of HBV infection.

13. All of the following are true regarding chronic hepatitis C except:

a) Acute infection goes onto chronic infection approximately 15-20% of the time.
b) Chronic infection leads to cirrhosis in 20-40% of cases.
c) Hep C patients with decompensated cirrhosis should not be treated with interferon but should be considered for liver transplantation.
d) Hepatitis A and B vaccines are recommended for all patients with Hep C.

14. The National Institute of Health recently came up with a series of guidelines for prevention of hepatitis C transmission. All of the following accurately convey a few of these guidelines except:

a) Since the risk of transmission is low (<3%) in monogamous long-term, no changes in sexual practices are recommended for these individuals.
b) Limiting close contact with family members and avoiding the sharing of meals or utensils is recommended.
c) Pregnancy is not contraindicated in women with HCV infection. The risk of transmission to the fetus is low (3-6%)
d) There is no evidence of transmission during breastfeeding; therefore, breast-feeding is considered safe and should be encouraged.

15. Each of the following is considered an extraintestinal manifestation of chronic hepatitis C infection except:

a) Porphyria cutanea tarda
b) Cryoglobulinemia, type II
c) Leukocytoclastic vasculitis
d) Focal segmental glomerulonephritis

16. All of the following are true regarding hepatitis E except:

a) Hepatitis E is an RNA virus that encodes just 3 genes.
b) Epidemiologically, hepatitis E resembles hepatitis B.
c) If a woman in her 3rd trimester acquires hep E, she bears a high risk of going onto fulminant hepatitis.
d) Hepatitis E occurs primarily in India, Asia, Africa, and Central America.

17. Each of the following are true for autoimmune hepatitis except:

a) One commonly sees ↑↑serum gamma globulins.
b) It affects primarily young women; average age 20-30 yo.
c) Labs may also show a + anti-Smooth muscle Ab.
d) Glucocorticoids are the mainstay of treatment.

18. All of the following are accurate statements regarding primary biliary cirrhosis except:
    a) PBC is an idiopathic disease of middle-aged women affecting the medium-to-large bile ducts.
    b) Labs that may be seen include an increased alk phos, increased IgM, and a + AMA (anti-mitochondrial antibody).
    c) Common symptoms include pruritis and steatorrhea (2° to progressive cholestasis).
    d) Ursodeoxycholic acid (UCDA) is currently viewed as an effective treatment for primary biliary cirrhosis (PBC).

19. All of the following accurately characterize primary sclerosing cholangitis except:
    a) It is felt to be autoimmune in origin.
    b) Ulcerative Colitis is associated in 70% of cases and almost uniformly precedes PSC.
    c) There is an increased risk of cholangiocarcinoma (bile duct ca).
    d) Treatment is primarily supportive, although many patients require liver transplant.

20. Oral contraceptives may lead to a variety of toxic effects on the liver. All of the following are examples of this except:
    a) Peliosis hepatis
    b) Adenomas ± intraperitoneal rupture
    c) Focal nodular hyperplasia
    d) Steatohepatitis

21. Peliosis hepatis (blood-filled cysts in the liver) is a complication associated with all of the following except:
    a) Pregnancy
    b) Vinyl chloride
    c) Anabolic steroids (also ↑ risk of angiosarcoma)
    d) Bartonella henselae (re: cause of cat-scratch disease and bacillary angiomatosis)

22. A number of disorders may be associated with hepatic vein thromboses. Among those, several are listed below. Find the exception:

    a) Inflammatory bowel disease
    b) Polycythemia vera
    c) Paroxysmal Nocturnal Hemoglobinuria
    d) Wilson's disease

23. An obese diabetic presents to your clinic with a recent history of an increase in her alcohol intake and periodic pain in her right upper quadrant. Exam is equivocal for hepatomegaly and there is no tenderness on your exam. LFTs reveal only a modest elevation of her aminotransferases. RUQ ultrasound reveals steatohepatitis. In addition to obesity, diabetes, and alcohol, all of the following may lead to steatohepatitis except:

a) Addison's syndrome
b) Pregnancy
c) Inflammatory bowel disease
d) Thyrotoxicosis

24. A 38 yo female presents with complaints of several months of solid and liquid food dysphagia that has been getting worse over the past month. Over the past month also she has noticed a new cough that usually occurs after meals. She has no complaints of heartburn and has suffered no weight loss. She has a normal skin exam. All of the following are manometric or radiographic features you might expect *except*:

a) Incomplete relaxation of the lower esophageal sphincter on manometry
b) Decreased amplitude or disappearance of peristaltic waves in the lower two-thirds of the esophagus on manometry
c) Tertiary contractions replacing peristaltic activity at all levels on manometry
d) A dilated esophagus with tapered lower end on upper GI

25. A 26 yo black male presents for the first time with complaints of intermittent diarrhea for several years, along with crampy abdominal pain, increased gas, and bowel movements that are loose. He denies any associated blood or fever or floating/excessively noxious stools. He thinks the symptoms are worse after he eats such foods as New England clam chowder, his morning cereal, and ice cream. The next best step in diagnoses would be:

a) Sudan stain for qualitative fecal fat
b) Checking the serum for anti-gliadin antibody
c) Testing for a positive hydrogen breath test following oral lactose
d) Lactose-free diet with follow-up in 2-3 weeks

26. All of the following are bacterial causes of bloody diarrhea except:

a) Yersinia enterocolytica
b) E. Coli 0157H7
c) Salmonella
d) Campylobacter jejuni

27. A patient with previously diagnosed systemic sclerosis presents for the first time with dysphagia to solids and liquids as well as severe reflux. All of the following upper GI findings would be consistent with this disorder except:

    a) Narrowing of the duodenum and jejunum
    b) Pseudoobstruction
    c) Common E-G tube
    d) Wide-mouthed jejunal diverticula

28. All of the following are true statements concerning Wilson's disease except:

    a) Coomb's negative hemolytic anemia can be seen in fulminant hepatitis.
    b) If a patient with frank neurologic or psychiatric disease does not have Kayser-Fleischer rings when examined by a trained observer using a slit lamp, the diagnosis of Wilson's disease can be excluded.
    c) Penicillamine and zinc, chelating agents, are generally lifelong and should be taken together whenever possible.
    d) Serum ceruloplasmin is decreased.

For questions # 29 through 35, match each medication with the hepatic disease it can either give or simulate. Choose the one BEST answer.

A. Viral hepatitis
B. Steatosis
C. Primary Biliary Cirrhosis
D. Granulomatous (hypersensitivity) hepatitis
E. Alcoholic liver disease (mimics)
F. Massive ischemic necrosis
G. Cholestatic jaundice

29. Allopurinol
30. Amiodarone
31. Amoxicillen-clavulinate; oral contraceptives
32. Chlorpromazine
33. Cocaine
34. Isoniazid
35. Tetracycline; AZT; valproic acid

36. Each of the following complications of ulcerative colitis are responsive to colectomy except:
    a) Sclerosing cholangitis
    b) Pyoderma gangrenosum
    c) Para-rectal disease
    d) Peripheral arthropathy

37. VIPoma is a tumor whose primary is usually in the pancreas, producing elevated levels of vasoactive intestinal peptide. This results in profuse, watery diarrhea and dehydration. In addition, which of the following signs is a feature of VIPoma?

a) Hypocalcemia
b) Colicky abdominal pain ("pancreatic cholera")
c) Achlorhydria
d) Hypokalemia

38. All of the following are features of glucagonoma, an alpha cell pancreatic tumor, except:

a) Stomatitis
b) Thromboembolism
c) Steatorrhea
d) Necrolytic migratory erythema

39. All of the following are true regarding the gastrinomas of Zollinger-Ellison Syndrome except:

a) If resection is curative, patients can expect a normal life expectancy. If not, average life expectancy is 7-10 years.
b) The gastrinomas yield ectopic G-cell hypersecretion.
c) The tumor is usually located in the pancreatic head.
d) Two-thirds of them are malignant, and ¼ of them are part of the MEN I syndrome.

40. Which of the following is an untrue statement regarding the secretory properties of gastrinomas in relationship to diagnosis and treatment?

a) A single duodenal ulcer is the most common radiographic finding in ZES.
b) One should suspect it in cases of recurrent, poorly responsive, or retrobulbar duodenal ulcers.
c) Serum fasting gastrin levels (>1200pg/ml) is the most sensitive and specific test, but it requires a low pH be present.
d) The secretin test can confirm the diagnosis by demonstrating an exaggerated decrease in gastrin level in response to infused secretin.

41. All of the following are features of carcinoid syndrome except:
a) Cor pulmonale
b) Endocardial fibrosis
c) Bradycardia
d) Asthma

42. Find the feature that is least likely to be true for a patient with diarrhea, flushing, facial edema and hypotension, and ascites.
    a) Elevated urinary 5-HIAA levels
    b) If the gut is clean, the bronchus and gonads are the next most likely places to turn up disease.
    c) Proctoscopy may reveal melanosis coli and loss of haustra.
    d) 90% of the primary tumors are found in the liver.

Questions # 43-47 are related to selected malabsorption disorders. Match each disorder with its treatment. Choose the one BEST answer.

A. Low-fat diet; fat-soluble vitamins
B. Address the causative disease
C. Medium-chain triglycerides, low-oxalate diet, parenteral nutrition prn
D. B12, folate, tetracycline
E. Initial course of IV antibiotics followed by 1year PO Bactrim ds bid or Cefixime 400mg qd

43. Tropical sprue
44. Whipple's disease
45. Short-gut syndrome
46. Lymphangiectasia
47. Abetalipoproteinemia

For questions # 48-53, match the diagnosis to the appropriate history of dysphagia, "A" through "F".

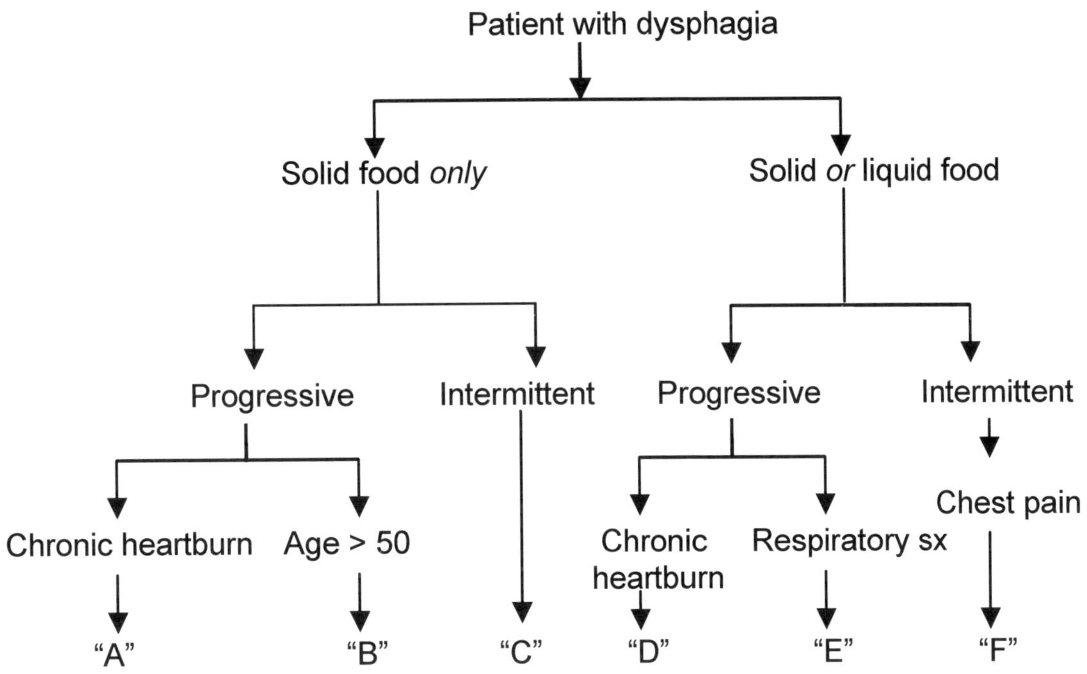

48. Achalasia
49. Carcinoma
50. Diffuse Esophageal Spasm
51. Lower esophageal ring
52. Peptic stricture
53. Scleroderma

54. All of the following are considered autoantibodies in celiac disease except:

    a) Anti-gluten antibody
    b) Anti-endomysial antibody
    c) Anti-gliadin antibody
    d) Anti-reticulin antibody

55. A 50 yo man presents with a history of steatorrhea, persistent non-specific GI upset and a bullous skin disease. His labs reveal Hgb of 10.2 g/dl and Hct of 30. MCV is 75. His labs are otherwise normal and except for a 10 lb weight loss from his last exam a year ago and the rash, physical exam is non-contributory. You tell him to avoid foods with wheat, rye, barley, oats, and malt. On follow-up exam 1 month later, he feels his steatorrhea has improved, though incompletely, and he complains of increased abdominal pain, nausea, and some low-grade fevers. He denies any chills or night sweats. Exam reveals an additional 3 lb weight loss. There is no hepato/splenomegaly and no palpable abdominal mass. The next best step in managing this patient is to rule out:

a) A secondary infectious intestinal disease
b) Whipple's disease
c) Intestinal lymphoma
d) Intestinal lymphangiectasia

56. All of the following are true regarding blind loop syndrome following gastrectomy except:

a) Bacterial overgrowth occurs in the afferent loop accounting for the clinical presentation.
b) Steatorrhea, microcytic anemia, weight loss, abdominal pain, and vitamin deficiencies are seen.
c) This syndrome is not the same as afferent loop syndrome.
d) Treatment is to convert the Bilroth II to Bilroth I or Roux-en-Y.

57. A 42 yo female presents with complaints of steatorrhea for 5 weeks along with an 8 lb weight loss. Her exam is essentially unrevealing. Her Sudan stain is positive, and a follow-up 72-hour quantitative fecal fat test yields 8grams. You order a D-Xylose test. All of the following are true regarding the workup of malabsorption in this patient except:

a) The purpose of the D-Xylose test is to show if the etiology is related to a mucosal lesion or bacterial overgrowth..
b) The ^{14}C-xylose breath test is not another name for the D-xylose test.
c) A positive ^{14}C-xylose is indicative of bacterial overgrowth.
d) The ^{14}C-xylose test works by measuring exhaled $^{14}CO_2$.

58. All of the following are true regarding the workup of pancreatic insufficiency except:
   a) A normal D-xylose test usually points to pancreatic insufficiency as the cause of malabsorption.
   b) The secretin and bentiromide tests are tests used to confirm pancreatic insufficiency.
   c) The secretin test is diagnostic of pancreatic exocrine insufficiency if there is a increase in pancreatic fluid output and bicarbonate secretion after an IV dose of secretin. This test is performed under fluoroscopic guidance.
   d) In testing with bentiromide (a synthetic peptide attached to PABA), chymotryspin cleaves the two and levels of arylamine (a biproduct of PABA) are measured in the urine; low levels are diagnostic of pancreatic insufficiency.

59. All of the following are considered factors in evaluating Ranson's criteria *at the time of admission or diagnosis* except:
   a) Hematocrit
   b) White blood cell count
   c) Glucose level
   d) Patient's age

60. All of the following are considered factors in evaluating Ranson's criteria *during the initial 48 hours* except:
   a) Serum calcium
   b) Change in blood urea nitrogen
   c) Lactate dehydrogenase
   d) Arterial pO_2

61. Each of the following is true regarding the potential complications of acute pancreatitis except:
   a) A phlegmon is a mass of inflamed pancreatic tissue.
   b) Pseudocysts are fluid collections that usually must be drained.
   c) Hypocalcemia is secondary to accumulation and/or precipitation of calcium salts.
   d) Pancreatic abscess usually occurs 2-4 weeks after the acute episode and may be recognized by a persistently elevated amylase.

62. All of the following medications are known for their ability to give a pancreatitis except:
   a) Pentamidine
   b) Furosemide
   c) Valproic acid
   d) Mezlocillin

63. All of the following are considered signs of pancreatic carcinoma if seen except:

   a) Courvoisier's sign
   b) Sentinel loop sign
   c) Trousseau's sign
   d) Double-duct sign

64. Each of the following is a characteristic of Whipple's disease except:

   a) Usually affects middle-aged men, but can affect either gender at any age
   b) May lead to hyperpigmentation
   c) Intestinal lymphoma is a potential complication
   d) May lead to heart failure and uveitis

Questions # 65-70 are matching-type questions regarding chronic gastritis, types A and B. Match all of the clinical associations with the correct type(s) of chronic gastritis.

A. Type A
B. Type B
C. Both types A and B
D. Neither type

65. Adenocarcinoma

66. Antrum of the stomach

67. Gastric carcinoids

68. H. Pylori (& PUD)

69. Increased serum gastrin

70. Pernicious anemia

71. Of the following, which is the least appropriate test to confirm eradication of H. Pylori one month after treatment?
   a) Urease Breath Test
   b) Antibody testing for H. Pylori with ELISA
   c) Stool antigen testing
   d) Endoscopic biopsy combined with the CLO test

Right- and left-sided diarrheas may have different presentations. For the following set of questions, match each characteristic to its correct side-predominance.

A. Right-sided diarrhea
B. Left-sided diarrhea

72. Anemia
73. Constipation/obstipation
74. Large volume stool
75. May note urgency, tenesmus, mucus, blood
76. Presentation more insidious

For the following set of questions, match each feature to the appropriate toxigenic or invasive bacterial diarrhea.

A. Staph aureus
B. Clostridium botulinum
C. Clostridium perfringes
D. E. Coli, enterotoxigenic
E. Vibrio cholerae
F. B. Cereus
G. Salmonella
H. Vibrio parahemolyticus
I. Yersinia enterocolytica
J. E. Coli 0157H7
K. Vibrio vulnificus
L. Campylobacter jejuni

77. "Church picnic"/buffet diarrhea; precooked foods; results from the survival of heat-resistant spores in inadequately cooked meat, poultry, or legumes

78. 2 forms: 1) skin/muscle inflammation /infection after exposure to seawater or cleaning fish; and 2) septicemia/necrotizing vasculitis/gangrene/shock after ingesting raw oysters

79. An invasive diarrhea with no fever; enterohemorrhagic; causative agent for hemolytic uremic syndrome

80. The emetic form of this food poisoning is associated with contaminated fried rice; the organism is common in uncooked rice, and its heat-resistant spores survive boiling. If cooked rice is not refrigerated, the spores can germinate and produce toxin. Frying before serving may not destroy the preformed, heat-stable toxin.

81. Differential diagnosis of its mesenteric adenitis includes acute appendicitis and Crohn's disease; iron overload states may predispose

82. May predispose to Guillain Barre syndrome; most common cause of bacterial enteritis

83. Neurotoxin interferes with presynaptic release, sometimes causing a descending paralysis

84. No antibiotics necessary unless + blood culture; usually no bloody diarrhea; eggs/poultry; fecal-oral route

85. Rapid onset (2-4h) after custard pastries or delicatessen meats

86. The only toxigenic bacterial diarrhea for which antibiotics have clearly been shown to decrease disease duration (tetracycline); treatment also decreases volume losses, and duration of excretion.

87. Undercooked shellfish, Chesapeake Bay; antibiotics do not decrease the course

88. Usually self-limiting; Cipro often taken prophylactically (prior to visiting parts of Mexico for example)

89. Campylobacter jejuni enteritis and ulcerative colitis share a number of potential features. All of the following are true statements except:

    a) Each commonly causes a bloody diarrhea.
    b) Both can cause toxic megacolon.
    c) Both are associated with arthritis.
    d) Patients with UC are predisposed to campylobacter infections.

90. Pseudoobstruction presents with clinical findings of mechanical obstruction but without occlusion of the lumen. All of the following may cause pseudoobstruction except:
    a) Amyloidosis
    b) Lorazepam
    c) Parkinson's disease
    d) Myxedema
    e) Hypoparathyroidism

For the following set of questions, match the features with the appropriate disease(s).

A. Ulcerative colitis
B. Crohn's disease
C. Both
D. Neither

91. Fibrosis

92. Granulomas

93. Malignancy (with long-standing disease)

94. Mesenteric fat/lymph node involvement

95. Palpable mass

96. Rectal bleeding

97. Recurrence after colectomy

98. Toxic megacolon

99. Several therapeutic agents in inflammatory bowel disease are used for colitis *maintenance* in ulcerative colitis and *active* colonic disease in Crohn's. Which one of the following medications is used for disease *maintenance* in both?

a) Mesalamine (Pentasa®)
b) Mesalamine (Asacol®)
c) Sulfasalazine (Azulfidine®)
d) Olsalazine (Dipentum®)

100. All of the following are true about inflammatory bowel disease except:

a) Rectal bleeding is more common in UC than in Crohn's.
b) Colonoscopy is contraindicated in acute UC secondary to the risk of perforation.
c) Among the extraintestinal manifestations of IBD, ankylosing spondylitis and sacroiliitis mirror the colitis.
d) In the setting of ileal disease and an intact colon, there is increased colonic absorption of dietary oxalate, with resulting hyperoxaluria and the development of urinary oxalate stones. Dehydration due to diarrhea is an additional predisposing factor in renal stone formation.

For the next set of questions on GI disease in AIDS, match the clinical description with the correct causative organism.

A. Histoplasmosis capsulatum
B. MAI
C. Cryptosporidium
D. Microsporidia
E. Isospora belli
F. Giardia lamblia
G. Blastocystis hominis
H. Cyclospora

101. Affects the small intestine, causing diarrhea; albendazole is the primary treatment of choice

102. Colonic involvement; treatment is amphotericin or itraconazole.

103. Diagnosis via oval oocysts in the stool seen with modified Kinyoun acid-fast stain. Primary treatment choice is TMP-SMX (160/800 mg qid for 10 days and then bid for 3 weeks) for treatment

104. Prominent early symptoms include diarrhea, abdominal pain, bloating, belching, flatus, nausea, and vomiting. Although diarrhea is common, upper intestinal manifestations such as nausea, vomiting, bloating, and abdominal pain may predominate. Associated with camping trips; "white-water rafting"; questions involving "Venezuela"(!); treatment is metronidazole.

105. Role as a pathogen is controversial; no controlled treatment trials.

106. Some patients may harbor the infection without symptoms, but many have diarrhea, flu-like symptoms, flatulence and burping. The diagnosis can be made by detection of spherical 8- to 10-um oocysts in the stool. These refractile oocysts are variably acid-fast and are fluorescent when viewed with ultraviolet light microscopy.

107. Voluminous diarrhea typically associated with fever, abdominal pain, and weight loss.

108. Voluminous, watery diarrhea. In immunocompromised hosts, especially those with AIDS, diarrhea can be chronic, persistent, and remarkably profuse, causing clinically significant fluid and electrolyte depletion. Stool volumes may range from 1 to 25 L/d; no therapy *proven* efficacious, although in AIDS patients, may try treating with paromomycin.

109. A patient with a history of long-standing history of coronary artery disease presents with severe abdominal pain , a single episode of hematochezia, and hypotension. Exam reveals only minimal nonfocal tenderness to palpation. Labs reveal an anion gap acidosis and an elevated leukocyte count of 16, 000. All of the following are true for this patient except:

a) Barium enema is hazardous in the acute situation because of the risk of perforation.
b) When thumbprinting is seen on plain films, it is often secondary to a thick, edematous bowel wall.
c) She should be scheduled for abdominal angiogram in the next hour.
d) Surgical resection may be required in some patients with fulminant ischemic colitis to remove gangrenous bowel.

110. Each of the following is considered an exudate on paracentesis except:

a) Meig's syndrome
b) Tuberculosis
c) Spontaneous Bacterial Peritonitis
d) Mesothelioma

111. All of the following are true for SBP (Spontaneous Bacterial Peritonitis) except:

a) Nearly always involves a single organism
b) 10-20% of patients with cirrhosis develop SBP
c) If suspect SBP and no extended-spectrum β-lactamases, patient should be started on a third generation cephalosporin or extended spectrum penicillin after cultures are obtained.
d) An ascitic fluid total leukocyte count of greater than 250 cells/uL (with a proportion of polymorphonuclear leukocytes of 50 percent or greater) should suggest the diagnosis of SBP.

112. All of the following appropriately describe features of hepatorenal syndrome except:

a) A serious complication in the patient with cirrhosis and ascites and is characterized by worsening azotemia with avid sodium retention and oliguria in the absence of identifiable specific causes of renal dysfunction.
b) Urinalysis and pyelography are usually normal.
c) The diagnosis is supported by the demonstration of marked urinary sodium retention. Typically, the urine sodium concentration is less than 5 mmol/L, much lower than that generally found in uncomplicated prerenal azotemia.
d) Worsening azotemia, hypernatremia, progressive oliguria, and hypertension are the hallmarks of the hepatorenal syndrome.

For the next set of questions match the current recommendation (from the revised ACS guidelines for screening and surveillance for colorectal polyps/cancer) with the correct risk category:

RISK CATEGORY	RECOMMENDATION	AGE TO BEGIN	INTERVAL
answer "A"	Colonoscopy	At the time of initial polyp diagnosis	TCE within 3y after initial polypectomy; if normal, TCE q5y
answer "B"	TCE	Age 40, or 10y before the youngest case in the family, whichever is earlier	Q5y
answer "C"	Colonoscopy and counseling to consider genetic testing	Age 21	If genetic test is + , or if patient has not had genetic testing, colonoscopy q2y until age 40, and then q year
answer "D"	Colonoscopies with biopsies for dysplasia	8 years after the start of pancolitis; 12-15 y after the start of L-sided colitis	Q1-2 y

DCBE=double-contrast barium enema; FOBT = fecal occult blood test; FS = flex sig; TCE = total colon examination

1. Digital rectal exam should be done at the time of each flex sig, colonoscopy, or DCBE.
2. Annual FOBT has been shown to reduce mortality from colorectal ca, so it is preferable to no screening.
3. TCE includes either DCBE or TCE.

113. Colorectal ca or adenomatous polyps in 1st degree relative <60 or in ≥2 first degree relatives of any age
114. Family h/o HNPCC
115. IBD
116. Large (≥1 cm) or multiple adenomatous polyps of any size

117. All of the following are true concerning colonic polyps except:
   a) Villous adenomas carry a greater risk of malignant transformation than do tubular adenomas
   b) Peutz-Jeghers is a polyposis syndrome of hamartomas in contrast to other heritable GI polyposis syndromes. The hamartomas have no increased risk of malignant transformation.
   c) Hyperplastic polyps are almost always benign.
   d) The likelihood that an adenoma which is 1.5-2.5cm in size will become malignant is on the order of 2-10%

118. AIDS cholangiopathy exhibits features similar to those found in primary sclerosing cholangitis and is typically associated with certain organisms. Of the following, which is *not* considered a key common cause of AIDS cholangiopathy?
   a) Cryptosporidia
   b) Microsporidia
   c) Giardia
   d) Cytomegalovirus

For the following set of questions, match each feature with the intestinal disease. Choose the one best answer.

A. Celiac disease
B. Crohn's disease
C. Ulcerative Colitis

119. Abdominal mass frequent
120. Bloody diarrhea common
121. Chronic cases carry the greatest risk for developing adenocarcinoma
122. Increased risk of developing intestinal lymphoma
123. Iron and B12 anemia
124. Iron and folate anemias
125. Mucosal 'cobblestone' lesions
126. Mucosal 'skip' lesions
127. Normal B12 absorption
128. Normal ESR
129. Perianal disease in most patients
130. Rectal involvement always
131. Strictures common

For this next set match each bacterial food poisoning with its correct pathogenesis. Choose the one best answer.

A. Staph aureus
B. Clostridium perfringes
C. Bacillus cereus
D. Clostridium botulinum

132. Enterotoxins
133. Ingestion of living organism
134. Spores produce a heat-labile neurotoxin
135. Mucosal invasion

For the next set of questions, match the pathological finding with the correct histological diagnosis of chronic hepatitis.

	Portal Inflammation	*Periportal Inflammation*	*Piecemeal Necrosis*	*Bridging Necrosis*	*Fibrosis*
A.	+	-	-	-	minimal
B.	+	minimal	scattered	-	some
C.	+	+	+	often	marked

136. Chronic active
137. Chronic lobular
138. Chronic persistent

139. All of the following are considered extra-hepatic features of autoimmune hepatitis except:
    a) Arthralgias
    b) Spider nevi
    c) Leukocytosis
    d) Amenorrhea
    e) Acne

140. From below, choose the correct assemblage of laboratory features in Wilson's disease.

	Ceruloplasmin	***Total Serum Copper***	***Urine Copper***	***Liver Cu***
a)	↑	↑	↑	↑
b)	↓	↑	↑	↑
c)	↓	↓	↑	↑
d)	↑	↓	↑	↑

141. Several of the hyperlipidemias are associated with acute pancreatitis. From greatest to least, what is the correct order of degree of association with acute pancreatitis.

a) Type V > I > IV
b) Type IV > V > I
c) Type IV > I > V
d) Type I > IV > V

INFECTIOUS DISEASES & HIV QUESTIONS

1. All of the following are true regarding the West Nile-like virus except:
   a) The virus is a mosquito-borne virus that can cause encephalitis and meningitis.
   b) It is spread to humans by the bite of a mosquito that becomes infected when feeding on infected birds.
   c) There is no evidence that the disease may spread from person to person.
   d) Individuals can contract the virus from handling an infected bird.
   e) For individuals who contract the virus, treatment is supportive and symptomatic only, and there is no directed therapy.

2. All of the following are true regarding EBV serology except:
   a) EA ('Early Antigen') 'D' component is a useful marker of current infection in patients who are EA +.
   b) VCA (viral capsid antigen) IgM is extremely useful in heterophile-negative cases for confirming acute disease.
   c) EBNA IgG indicates prior infection and persists for up to 1 year following infection.
   d) EBNA (EBV-associated nuclear antigen) indicates infected cells harboring viral genome.

3. All of the following reflect true statements regarding the pattern of spread in Varicella-Zoster Virus except:
   a) Reactivation of latent VZV is most common after the sixth decade of life in non-immunosuppressed individuals.
   b) Varicella pneumonia is the most serious complication following chickenpox, developing more commonly in adults (up to 20 percent of cases) than in children.
   c) Most patients with zoster have no history of recent exposure to other individuals with VZV infection.
   d) Patients who have never had chicken pox can get zoster by exposure to someone with shingles.
   e) Patients who have never had chicken pox can get chicken pox by exposure to someone with shingles.

4. All of the following are clinical associations with Parvovirus B19 except:
   a) Erythema infectiosum
   b) Transient aplastic crisis
   c) Asymmetric migratory polyarthropathy
   d) Chronic anemia in immunodeficient patients
   e) Fetal and congenital infection

5. All of the following are true regarding rotavirus infections except:
   a) It causes a watery diarrheal illness in children.
   b) It is frequently contracted through swimming pools primarily in the summer.
   c) It is diagnosed via stool antigen using the ELISA technique.
   d) Treatment is symptomatic only.

6. All of the following are clinical associations with Human Papilloma Virus except:
   a) Plantar warts
   b) Flat warts
   c) Condyloma acuminata
   d) Oral hairy leukoplakia
   e) Skin squamous cell carcinoma in transplant patients

7. All of the following are true regarding rabies except:
   a) Direct Fluorescent Antibody testing may be done on skin obtained by biopsy from the back of the neck.
   b) HRIG (Human Rabies Immune Globulin) *plus* vaccine plays an important role if given within the first 10 days of symptom onset.
   c) Half of the HRIG should be injected *directly* into the wound and the rest into the *gluteal* area.
   d) In rabies post-exposure prophylaxis, following an animal bite from rodents, squirrels, or mice, patients almost never require anti-rabies vaccine.

8. Each of the following regarding Rubella and pregnancy is a true statement except:
   a) Pregnant women should not be given the vaccine since it may cause congenital defects.
   b) Women of child-bearing age should be warned not to become pregnant for 2-3 months following vaccination.
   c) If a pregnant woman's rubella titre shows non-immune, it should be rechecked 2-3 weeks later. If it hasn't increased, no treatment is necessary.
   d) If the pregnant woman is non-immune and is rechecked 2-3 weeks later and has seroconverted, she should be considered for early C-section delivery to avoid complications regarding delivery.

Questions # 9-12 are matching-type questions on Hepatitis B post-exposure prophylaxis. Match the appropriate post-exposure prophylaxis recommendation to the situation, A, B, C, or D.

EXPOSED PATIENT	EXPOSURE SOURCE	
	HBsAg +	**HBsAg -**
Unvaccinated	"A"	"B"
Vaccinated	"C"	"D"

9. No treatment
10. Vaccine only
11. HBIG + vaccine
12. If exposed person has anti-HBs $\geq$ 10, $\rightarrow$No treatment. If < 10, $\rightarrow$HBIG + 1 dose of vaccine.

13. Of the following choices, which is the closest meaning to the meaning of "triple therapy" in HIV?
    a) Two non-nucleoside analogues plus one protease inhibitor
    b) One nucleoside analogue plus one non- nucleoside analogue plus one protease inhibitor
    c) Two nucleoside analogues plus either one non-nucleoside analogue or one protease inhibitor.
    d) Two non-nucleoside analogues plus one protease inhibitor

14. Which of the following nucleoside analogues (reverse transcriptase inhibitors) is a frequent cause of hypertriglyceridemia?
    a) Abacavir
    b) Stavudine
    c) Didanosine
    d) Lamivudine

15. Choose from among the following statements, regarding HIV therapy, the statement that is *least* likely to be true.
    a) Patients being treated for PCP (pneumocystis carinii pneumonia) with TMP-SMX have a reduced frequency of toxoplasmosis.
    b) Patients who are being treated with sulfadiazene-pyrimethamine are protected against PCP and do not need additional prophylaxis against PCP.
    c) Rifampin should not be administered concurrently with nucleoside reverse transcriptase inhibitors. Rifabutin should be used instead.
    d) PCP prophylaxis may be discontinued if the CD4 $\geq$200 for $\geq$ 3-6 months.

16. Of the choices below, which are the appropriate indications for glucocorticoid use in pneumocystis carinii pneumonia?
    a) PaO_2 < 70 or A-a gradient >35
    b) Bilateral interstitial infiltrates with history of dyspnea on exertion
    c) Bilateral interstitial infiltrates with evidence of desaturation on exercise
    d) PaO_2 <90 or an O2 saturation <93%

17. All of the following are true regarding infections from pseudomonas aeruginosa except:
    a) It is a common organism complicating burns.
    b) It causes malignant otitis externa in diabetics.
    c) It commonly causes ecthyma gangrenosum in CLL patients.
    d) Colonization with P. aeruginosa correlates with bronchial airway disease in cystic fibrosis patients.

In the prophylaxis of opportunistic disease in HIV, there are a number of important drug-drug interactions to be aware of. For the following set of questions, choose whether the level of the drug affected goes up or down. Choose "A" for up or "B" for down.

A. Affected drug level ↑ by culprit drug
B. Affected drug level ↓ by culprit drug

QUESTION	AFFECTED DRUG	CULPRIT DRUG
#18.	Atovaquone	Rifampin
#19.	Clarithromycin	Ritonavir
#20.	Clarithromycin	Nevirapine
#21.	Ketoconazole	Antacids, didanosine (ddI), H2-receptor antagonists, proton-pump inhibitors
#22.	Quinolone antibiotics	Didanosine, antacids, iron products, calcium products, sucralfate
#23.	Rifabutin	Fluconazole
#24.	Rifabutin	Efavirenz
#25.	Rifabutin	Ritonavir, saquinavir, indinavir, nelfinavir, amprenavir, delavirdine

For the following set of questions match each medication used in the treatment of HIV disease to the side effect of greatest clinical import from among the following choices. Choose the one BEST answer.

A. Anemia
B. GI upset, pancreatitis, peripheral neuropathy
C. Neuropathy
D. Hypertriglyceridemia
E. Rash (possibly severe life-threatening, e.g. Stevens-Johnson syndrome or TEN)
F. Altered mental status
G. GI upset, paresthesias
H. Nephrolithiasis
I. Nausea
J. Diarrhea

26. Abacavir (ABC) (Ziagen)
27. Amprenavir (Agenerase)
28. Didanosine (ddI) (Videx)
29. Efavirenz (Sustiva)
30. Indinavir (Crixivan)
31. Nelfinavir (Viracept)
32. Nevirapine (Viramune)
33. Ritonavir (Norvir)

34. Saquinavir (Fortovase)
35. Stavudine (d4T) (Zerit)
36. Zalcitabine (ddC) (Hivid)
37. Zidovidine (AZT) (Retrovir)

38. Each of the following is true about chlamydia psittacosis except:
    a) Transmitted from asymptomatic avian carriers pet-shop owners, poultry workers, pigeon fanciers, taxidermists, veterinarians, and zoo attendants.
    b) Clinical presentation includes fever, chills, headache, productive cough, and stiff neck.
    c) Alveolar macrophages containing characteristic cytoplasmic inclusion bodies. [Levinthal-Coles-Lillie (LCL) bodies] are pathognomonic of psittacosis.
    d) Symptoms of upper respiratory tract infection are not prominent.

39. Of the following statements regarding cat and dog bites, which is the least true?
    a) Cat bites are the most common form of transmission of pasteurella multocida.
    b) Capnocytophaga (formerly DF-2) is a more common pathogen in dog bites than in cat bites.
    c) Amoxicillin is a reasonable first choice for antibiotic coverage in dog or cat bites.
    d) Capnocytophaga commonly causes infection in splenectomized individuals, especially in alcoholics and immunosuppressed.

40. A comparison of cat scratch disease (CSD) and bacillary angiomatosis (BA) reveals all of the following except:
    a) CSD affects primarily immunosuppressed individuals vs. BA, which is more common in the immunocompetent.
    b) The organisms in both CSD and BA include bartonella henselae.
    c) CSD is self-limited while BA tends to be progressive/recurrent.
    d) Acquisition of B. henselae has been significantly associated with exposure to young cats infested with fleas.

41. All of the following are features associated with listeria monocytogenes infections except:
    a) Causes aseptic meningitis/bacteremia in neonates, immunosuppressed (e.g. lymphoma) and pregnant women
    b) Associated with consumption of contaminated milk, ice cream, undercooked hot dogs
    c) Although the prevalence of listeriosis among persons infected with human immunodeficiency virus (HIV) is much lower than that of the general population, listeriosis is a relatively common opportunistic infection in HIV.
    d) Recent studies of clinical series have shown that bacteremic infection without an evident focus is the most common clinical manifestation of listeriosis among immunocompromised hosts.

42. All of the following statements are true concerning neisseria gonorrhea and chlamydia trachomatis except:

    a) In patients with recurrent neisseria infections, CH50 is used to screen for terminal complement deficiencies.
    b) Approximately two-thirds of patients with disseminated gonococcal infection are men
    c) Gonococcal isolates from homosexual men tend to be more resistant to antimicrobials than are isolates from heterosexuals.
    d) Spread of gonococci or chlamydiae into the upper abdomen may cause perihepatitis (Fitz-Hugh-Curtis syndrome), manifested by right upper quadrant or bilateral upper-abdominal pain and tenderness and occasionally by a hepatic friction rub.

43. Regarding neisseria meningitidis, find the statement that is least accurate:

    a) The classic presentation is fever, hypotension, DIC, and purpura fulminans.
    b) Any febrile patient with a petechial rash should have blood cultures taken and treatment begun after the first cultures have returned.
    c) A single dose of Cipro 500mg PO is an appropriate choice of post-exposure prophylaxis.
    d) The nasopharynx is the natural habitat of meningococcus.

44. All of the following are true regarding brucellosis infections except:

    a) Brucella is transmitted most commonly through the ingestion of untreated milk or milk products, raw meat, or bone marrow and cannot be contracted via inhalation during contact with animals.
    b) Persons at risk include farmers, dairy workers; livestock handlers; meat packers; veterinary surgeons; and those who ingest unpasteurized dairy products.
    c) Brucella melitensis (the most common form worldwide) is acquired primarily from goats, sheep, and camels.
    d) Brucellae are killed by boiling or pasteurization of milk and milk products.

45. Each of the following is associated with Mycoplasma Pneumoniae except:

    a) Cold-agglutinin formation $\pm$ hemolytic anemia
    b) Erythema marginatum and the Stevens-Johnson syndrome
    c) Guillain Barre syndrome
    d) Mononeuritis multiplex

46. Actinomyces israelii is an anaerobic, gram +, branching, filamentous bacterium with all of the following potential features except:

    a) Paramandibular infection with a chronic draining sinus commonly preceded by an upper respiratory infection.
    b) Chest wound infection
    c) Marked cortical hypertrophy of the facial/jaw bones
    d) Pulmonary abscess

47. All of the following Rickettsial infections have an insect vector except:

    a) Erlichiosis
    b) Q fever
    c) Rocky Mountain Spotted Fever
    d) Endemic (murine) and epidemic typhus

48. All of the following Rickettsial infections typically yield a rash except:

    a) Scrub typhus and rickettsialpox
    b) Endemic (murine) and epidemic typhus
    c) Rickettsia prowazekii
    d) Q fever and erlichiosis

48. All of the following statements are true for Rocky Mountain Spotted Fever except:

    a) Erythematous and hemorrhagic macules and papules begin peripherally. (wrists/forearms, ankles) and spread centripetally (to arms, thighs, trunk, face).
    b) Fever, headache, myalgia are common symptoms. The rash usually begins on the 4th day of the fever.
    c) RMSF is seen throughout the Western border of the Rocky Mountains. A history of tick bite is given in 12% of cases.
    d) ↓Na+ is seen in half the cases.

50. Of the following, choose the statement that is least accurate regarding Erlichiosis:

    a) Morulae (Latin for “mulberry”: the appearance of the cytoplasmic inclusion, a vacuolar cluster of Giemsa-stained ehrlichiae in phagocytes) are frequently seen in the *granulocytic* type.
    b) Laboratories show ↓WBC, ↑platelets, and ↑LFTs.
    c) It is more common in spring and summer
    d) Also referred to as “Spotless Rocky Mountain Spotted Fever”

For the following set of questions, match each disease to the insect vector. Choose the one BEST answer.

A. *Ixodes dammini (deer ticks)*
B. *Dermacentor variabilis* (American dog tick)
C. *Liponyssoides sanguineus (mouse mite)*
D. Cat fleas
E. Human body louse (*Pediculus humanus corporis*)

51. Human Granulocytic Erlichiosis
52. Human Monocytic Erlichiosis
53. Lyme Disease
54. Rocky Mountain Spotted Fever (Eastern 2/3rds of the US and California)
55. Rickettsialpox
56. Endemic (murine) typhus
57. Epidemic typhus

58. All of the following are gram positive bacilli except:
    a) Brucella
    b) Corynebacterium
    c) Actinomyces israelii
    d) Listeria monocytogenes

59. In regards to enterococcus, all of the following are true except:
    a) PCN is bacteriastatic, not bacteriacidal against enterococci.
    b) Enterococci are generally resistant to all cephalosporins.
    c) Because of evidence of prolonged tissue infectivity with E. faecium, benzathine PCN G is the preferred initial treatment.
    d) E. faecalis is sensitive to PCN G. Gentamycin may be added for endocarditis or meningitis infections.

60. All of the following are true regarding clinical correlations of β-hemolytic group A streptococcal infections except:
    a) Untreated β-hemolytic group A strep pharyngitis predisposes to development of rheumatic fever
    b) β-hemolytic group A strep throat and skin infections predispose to post-streptococcal glomerulonephritis
    c) Immunofluorescence microscopy reveals diffuse granular deposition of IgG and C3, giving rise to a "starry sky" appearance.
    d) Prompt antibiotic therapy appears to prevent the development of post-streptococcal glomerulonephritis as well as rheumatic fever following throat infection.

61. Each of the following Jones criteria are considered major criteria except:
    a) Increase in ASO (anti-streptolysin-O) titre
    b) EKG changes
    c) Subcutaneous nodules
    d) Erythema marginatum

62. Concerning rheumatic fever, all of the following are true except:
    a) Clinical manifestations usually appear many years after the onset of pharyngitis.
    b) Cardiac damage is the only potentially chronic debilitating effect.
    c) Migratory polyarthritis occurs in about 70% of patients, characteristically shows rapid relief with ASA (usually within 48h) and never causes permanent joint damage.
    d) Treatment is with a complete 10-day course in adults of either oral penicillin V (500 mg twice daily), or erythromycin (250 mg four times daily) if pen-allergic.

For the following set of questions match each of the quinolone antibiotics to the appropriate antimicrobial spectrum or generation. Choose one best answer from either A, B, C, or D.

CLASSIFICATION OF QUINOLONE ANTIBIOTICS:		
Classification	Agent	Antimicrobial spectrum
First generation	Answer "A"	Gram-negatives (but no Pseudomonas)
Second generation	Answer "B"	Gram-negatives (including Pseudomonas), some gram + (Staph aureus but not Strep pneumoniae) and some atypicals
Third generation	Answer "C"	Same as for 2nd gen plus expanded gram + coverage (Pen-sensitive and Pen-resistant Strep pneumoniae) + expanded activity vs. atypicals
Fourth generation	Answer "D"	Same as for 3rd gen + broad anaerobic coverage

63. Cinoxacin (Cinobac)
64. Ciprofloxacin (Cipro)
65. Enoxacin (Penetrex)
66. Gatifloxacin (Tequin)
67. Levofloxacin (Levaquin)

68. Lomefloxacin (Maxaquin)
69. Moxifloxacin (Avelox)
70. Nalidixic acid (NegGram)
71. Norfloxacin (Noroxin)
72. Ofloxacin (Floxin)
73. Sparfloxacin (Zagam)
74. Trovafloxacin (Trovan)

75. A 33 yo woman presents following a bicycle accident in which she sustained a single dirty abrasion. She relates a history of two prior tetanus immunizations. What is the most appropriate recommendation regarding tetanus prophylaxis in her wound management?

    a) Cleanse the wound thoroughly with soap and water; bacitracin; and a gauze wrap. No additional passive or active immunization is necessary.
    b) After appropriate wound care, she should receive a third dose of Td only.
    c) After appropriately treating her wound, she should receive Td in addition to tetanus immune globulin.
    d) After appropriate wound care, she should receive tetanus immune globulin, since she has already had 2 prior Td vaccinations.

For the following set of questions, match each vaccine with its correct classification.

A. Toxoids
B. Recombinant vaccine
C. Pooled surface proteins
D. Attenuated (live) organism
E. Inactivated (killed) organism

76. BCG
77. Botulism
78. Cholera
79. Diphtheria
80. H. Flu B (HiB)
81. Hep A
82. Hep B
83. Influenza B
84. M, M, and R (all three)
85. Oral polio vaccine
86. Pertussis
87. Rabies
88. Strep Pneumococcus
89. Tetanus
90. Typhoid
91. VZV (Varicella-Zoster)
92. Yellow fever

93. None of the following conditions or procedures require endocarditis prophylaxis except:

a) Atrial septal defect, secundum
b) Permanent pacemaker
c) Transesophageal echocardiogram
d) Sclerotherapy of esophageal varices

94. All of the following conditions or procedures require endocarditis prophylaxis except:

a) Idiopathic hypertrophic subaortic stenosis
b) Rigid bronchoscopy
c) Cystoscopy
d) Routine cavity filling with local anesthetic

95. All of the following are considered indications for surgery in infective endocarditis except:

a) Severe reactive thrombocytosis
b) Refractory CHF
c) Prosthetic valve involvement
d) Hemolysis

For the following set of questions, match each situation with the organism that is most likely to cause endocarditis from among the choices given. Choose one BEST answer. Answers may be used more than once.

A. Strep viridans
B. Staph aureus
C. Staph epidermidis
D. Strep bovis

96. Colorectal carcinoma

97. IVDA

98. Native valves

99. Previous rheumatic valve damage

100. Prosthetic heart valve

For the following set of questions, match each scenario with the appropriate treatment for endocarditis, assuming the patient has no known drug allergies.

A. Pen G ± Gentamycin
B. Treatment depends on resistance to Pen/Aminoglycosides/Vanco
C. Nafcillin/Oxacillin + Gentamycin
D. Vancomycin
E. Ceftriaxone
F. Pen/Amp/Nafcillin/Oxacillin + Gent
G. Vanco + Gent + Rifampin
H. Vanco + Gent

101. Empiric therapy for native valve endocarditis
102. Empiric therapy for prosthetic valve endocarditis
103. Enterococci, native valve
104. HACEK organisms (fastidious, slow-growing gram-negative bacteria)
105. MRSA, native valve
106. MRSA, prosthetic valve
107. MSSA (Methicillin-sensitive staph aureus), native valve
108. MSSA, prosthetic valve
109. Staph epidermidis, prosthetic valve
110. Strep viridans, native valve

111. All of the following have clearly been shown to be involved in post-splenectomy infections except:
    a) Capnocytophaga
    b) Babesiosis
    c) Salmonella typhi
    d) N. meningitides

112. All of the following are potential findings on peripheral blood smear reflecting the chronic manifestations of splenectomy except:
    a) Marked variation in size and shape of erythrocytes (anisocytosis, poikilocytosis)
    b) Morulae formation
    c) Howell-Jolly bodies (nuclear remnants)
    d) Heinz bodies (denatured hemoglobin)
    e) Basophilic stippling
    f) Pappenheimer bodies

For the following questions, match each sexually transmitted disease to the latest recommended treatment. Choose the one BEST answer.

STD	TREATMENT GUIDELINES
"A"	Azithromycin single dose of 1g PO; or Ceftriaxone 250mg IM x1; or Erythro 500 qid x 1 week
"B"	Azithromycin single dose of 1g PO; or Doxy 100 BID x 1 week
"C"	Cipro 500 PO x1 or Ofloxacin 400 PO x1 or Ceftriaxone 125 IM x 1 or Cefixime 400 PO x 1
"D"	Doxycycline 100 BID x 3 weeks
"E"	Metronidazole 2g PO x 1; contraindicated in the 1st trimester pregnancy

113. Chancroid
114. Chlamydia trachomatis
115. GC, uncomplicated
116. Lymphogranuloma Venereum (LGV)
117. Trichomonas vaginalis

118. A 69 yo male presents 1 week following a transurethral resection of the prostate with left-sided scrotal pain, fever, and tenderness at the inferoposterior aspect of the left testes on examination. He denies any dysuria or hematuria. Urinalysis detects midstream pyuria only. A doppler flow study reveals no evidence of torsion or mass. Of the following, which would be the most appropriate treatment?
   a) Ciprofloxacin 500mg PO or ofloxacin 400mg bid x 10-14d
   b) Ceftriaxone 125 mg intramuscularly
   c) Ceftriaxone 250mg IM x 1 + doxy 100 mg po bid x 10d or ofloxacin 300mg po bid x 10d
   d) Immediate surgery

119. All of the following are true about granuloma inguinale except:
   a) Donovan bodies are commonly seen on microscopy.
   b) Calymmatobacterium granulomatis is the causative organism.
   c) Treatment is very similar to lymphogranuloma venereum.
   d) Granuloma inguinale is much more common among women, especially caucasian.

For the following set of questions, match each sexually transmitted disease with its causative organism.

A. Lymphogranuloma venereum (LGV)
B. Chancroid
C. Granuloma inguinale

120. Calymmatobacterium granulomatis
121. Chlamydia trachomatis
122. Hemophilus ducreyii

123. All of the following are true regarding aminoglycoside toxicity except:

a) Hypermagnesemia is a fairly common aminoglycoside toxicity.
b) The nephrotoxicity is almost always reversible.
c) NSAIDs, vanco, and ampho all can enhance aminoglycoside-induced nephrotoxicity.
d) The ototoxicity is almost always irreversible.

124. Which is the most appropriate initial antifungal management in an immunocompetent patient with primary pulmonary coccidioidomycosis?

a) Itraconazole or Ampho B
b) Fluconazole
c) Ampho B + Flucytosine
d) Antifungal treatment not necessary, but patient should be monitored periodically and treated if fever/weight loss/fatigue do not resolve within a month or two.

125. Which of the following are transmitted via bird droppings?

a) Coccidioides immitus
b) Histoplasmsosis
c) Blastomycosis
d) Cryptococcus neoformans
e) a & c
f) b & d
g) a, c, & d
h) All of the above

126. A 22 yo previously well-controlled asthmatic male presents with complaints of breakthrough wheezing and coughing up brown mucus plugs. Sputum culture is positive for aspergillus and IgE is >1000. Peripheral blood eosinophils are 1200. Medical records reveal a history of aspergillus 3 years ago on a sputum culture. The next best step in managing this patients is:

a) Initiate steroid therapy
b) Initiate double coverage for pseudomonas aeruginosa
c) Initiate antifungal therapy for allergic bronchopulmonary aspergillosis
d) No therapy necessary since aspergillus is a frequent colonizer of the respiratory tract

127. All of the following are true regarding sporotrichosis except:
  a) The causative organism is Sporothrix schenkii, a fungus commonly found in the soil.
  b) There are 2 main forms of skin disease: chronic lymphangitic and chancriform.
  c) Lugal solution (saturated solution of potassium iodide) is the primary drug of choice for cutaneous/lymphonodular involvement.
  d) Itraconazole is the drug of choice for osteoarticular arthritis.

128. Itraconazole is the primary antifungal of choice for all of the following except:
  a) Mild to moderate blastomycosis
  b) Coccidioidomycosis meningitis
  c) Moderate histoplasmosis in an immunocompetent individual
  d) Sporotrichosis

129. All of the following are true regarding mucormycosis except:
  a) Caused by Rhizopus, Zygomycetes
  b) Diagnosis based on finding black, necrotic lesions around the eyes, nose, soft/hard palates; a sharply delineated area of necrosis, strictly respecting the midline, may appear in the hard palate.
  c) Diabetics in ketoacidosis can develop rhinocerebral infections and coma, if seen, is usually due to the marked acidosis.
  d) Ampho B + surgical debridement

130. Each of the following is an accurate statement regarding toxoplasmosis except:
  a) It can present with a mononucleosis-like syndrome in the immunocompetent host.
  b) Brain lesions can be difficult to differentiate from CNS lymphoma, as both give ring-enhancing lesions.
  c) Acute toxoplasma infection evokes a cascade of protective immune responses in the normal host. Toxoplasma enters the host at the gut mucosal level and evokes the production of IgM antibody. Titers of serum IgM antibody directed at p30 (SAG-1) have been shown to be a useful marker of congenital and acute toxoplasmosis.
  d) The ingestion of a single cyst is all that is required for human infection. Undercooking or insufficient freezing of meat is an important source of infection in the developed world. In the United States, 10 to 20 percent of lamb products and 25 to 35 percent of pork products show evidence of cysts that contain bradyzoites.

131. Which of the following, when seen, is a poor prognosticator in malaria?
   a) Anemia
   b) Splenomegaly
   c) Hemoglobinuria
   d) Low glucose

For the following set of questions match each species of malaria with the primary treatment of choice. Each answer may be chosen once, more than once, or not at all.

A. Chloroquine
B. Chloroquine + Primaquine
C. Quinine sulfate + Doxycycline
D. Mefloquine
E. IV Quinidine
F. Doxycycline
G. None of the above

132. Plasmodium vivax
133. P. ovale
134. P. falciparum, chloroquine-sensitive
135. P. falciparum, chloroquine-resistant
136. P. malariae

137. The following are all true statements regarding malaria prophylaxis and recommendations except:
   a) Chloroquine is the first choice: 500mg PO q week, starting 1-2 weeks prior to travel and stopping 4 weeks after return.
   b) Mefloquine is indicated for chloroquine-resistant areas and is contraindicated in patients taking calcium channel blockers
   c) Doxycycline is indicated for chloroquine & mefloquine-resistant areas
   d) Patient should be advised to take 3 tabs at once of pyrimethamine-sulfadoxine should fever develop in areas endemic for malaria.

DERMATOLOGY QUESTIONS

Skin disease is often a manifestation of malignancy. For the following set of questions, match all of the skin diseases with the associated malignancy. Answers can be used only once.

A. Ovarian carcinoma
B. Glucagonoma
C. Sezary syndrome
D. Lung carcinoma
E. Multiple myeloma with 2° amyloidosis
F. Hodgkin's disease
G. Breast carcinoma
H. AML
I. Thymoma

1. Acanthosis nigricans
2. Acquired ichthyosis
3. Dermatomyositis
4. Erythema gyratum repens
5. Erythroderma
6. Necrolytic migratory erythema
7. Pemphigus
8. Post-proctoscopic periorbital pinch purpura
9. Sweet's syndrome

In internal medicine systemic disease often manifests with cutaneous signs. For the next set of questions, match the dermatologic manifestation to its systemic disease. Choose one best answer. Answers may be used only once.

A. Sarcoidosis
B. Lofgren's syndrome
C. Pseudoxanthoma elasticum
D. Zinc deficiency
E. Celiac disease
F. Reiter's syndrome
G. Atheroemboli
H. Scleroderma
I. Diabetes mellitus

10. Acrodermatitis enteropathica
11. Apthous ulcers
12. Dermatitis herpetiformis
13. E. Nodosum, fever, arthralgias, bilateral hilar lymphadenopathy
14. Livedo reticularis
15. Lupus Pernio
16. Morphea
17. Necrobiosis lipoidica diabeticorum
18. Yellow papules seen on the abdomen/groin/neck/axilla; angioid streaks in the retina

For the next set of questions match each description with the most likely diagnosis.

A. Toxic Epidermolysis Necrosis
B. Stevens-Johnson Syndrome
C. Staphylococcal Scalded Skin Syndrome
D. Toxic Shock Syndrome

19. A staph aureus toxin-mediated illness which causes fever, hypotension, generalized skin and mucosal erythema, and multisystem failure and occurs in menstrual and nonmenstrual forms.

20. A staph aureus toxin-mediated painful, tender, diffuse erythema typically followed by desquamation and occurring mainly in newborns and infants under 2 yo.

21. Considered a maximal variant of erythema multiforme; frequent culprits include allopurinol, aminopenicillins, and sulfa.

22. Mucocutaneous, usually drug-induced skin tenderness and erythema that is typically followed by extensive cutaneous and mucosal exfoliation. Considered a maximal variant of Stevens-Johnson syndrome.

For the following set of questions, match each description with the appropriate dermatologic disease.

A. Measles
B. Rocky Mt. Spotted Fever
C. Ecthyma gangrenosum
D. Impetigo
E. Erysipelas
F. Erysipeloid
G. Scarlet fever
H. Purpura fulminans
I. Cat scratch disease
J. Rosacea
K. Pityriasis versicolor
L. Pityriasis rosacea

23. A cellulitis with necrosis related to septic vasculitis. It begins with cutaneous infarction and progresses to larger, ulcerated lesions. The causative organism is Pseudomonas Aeruginosa; the patient is usually immunocompromised/ neutropenic and bacteremia is common

24. A chronic disorder of the facial pilosebaceous units. ↑ capillary sensitivity to heat results in flushing and ultimately telangiectasia

25. A chronic, asymptomatic scaling rash, characterized by well-demarcated scaling patches with variable hyperpigmentation, usually occurring on the trunk

26. A maculopapular rash that spreads from the head down and resolves in the same order after approximately 3 days

27. A violaceous erythematous cellulitis to the hand 2° to erysipelothrix rhusiopathiae after handling saltwater fish, shellfish, meat, hides, poultry

28. A benign, self-limiting infection characterized by a primary skin or conjunctival lesion and caused by the organisms formerly called Rochalimaea henselae.

29. Crusted golden-yellow erosions which become confluent on the nose, cheeks, chin, and lips secondary to Staph Aureus and Group A Strep (Pyogenes)

30. Desquamation + 'strawberry' tongue secondary to Group A Strep. Of note, Kawasaki disease is another disease that may give a strawberry tongue and a desquamating rash.

31. Distinctive rash that begins as a "herald patch", usually on the trunk, followed 1-2 weeks later with a generalized exanthematous eruption that resolves spontaneously after 6 weeks without therapy. More common in the spring and fall. May be 2° to picornavirus.

32. Erythematous and hemorrhagic macules and papules begin peripherally (wrists/forearms, ankles) and spread centripetally to arms, thighs, trunk, and face. Fever, headache, myalgia typically accompany.

33. The cutaneous manifestation of DIC in acute meningococcemia

34. Red, painful cellulitis 2° to Staph aureus, but more commonly group A Strep. The margins of the cellulitis are raised, and the borders are sharply demarcated.

35. All of the following are true concerning oral leukoplakia except:
    a) It is related to the Epstein Barr Virus.
    b) It is also associated with smoking, smokeless tobacco, alcohol, and syphilis.
    c) Candida can invade secondarily.
    d) It is considered a premalignant lesion for squamous cell carcinoma.

36. All of the following are true for basal cell carcinoma except:
    a) It is the most common type of skin cancer.
    b) The most common is noduloulcerative BCC, which begins as a small, pearly nodule, often with small telangiectatic vessels on its surface.
    c) Similar to squamous cell carcinoma, not only is sun exposure important in the development of the lesion, but arsenic exposure may also predispose.
    d) Unlike squamous cell carcinoma, basal cell ca has a high metastatic potential.

For the following set of questions, match each mucosal or cutaneous disease with the HPV serotypes most commonly associated. Choose one best answer "A" through "K".

MUCOSAL		CUTANEOUS	
6,11	A	1	E
34,40,42	B	2	F
72,73	C	3	G
16,18,31,33	D	5,8	H
		36	I
		48	J
		49	K

37. Actinic keratoses
38. Anogenital malignancies
39. Anogenital warts
40. Benign warts
41. Common warts
42. Flat warts
43. Genital warts
44. Intraepithelial neoplasia
45. Oral papillomas in immunosuppressed pts
46. Plantar warts
47. Squamous cell ca
48. Squamous cell carcinoma
49. Warts, actinic keratoses

50. Drug-induced erythroderma (exfoliative dermatitis), which often begins as a morbilliform rash, is known to be a fairly common skin reaction in all of the following except:
    a) Penicillins
    b) Sulfonamides
    c) Verapamil
    d) Carbamazepine
    e) Allopurinol

51. All of the following are true statements regarding HANE (hereditary angioneurotic edema) except:
    a) Lesions are typically quite pruritic and respond rapidly to administration of epinephrine.
    b) Levels of C1 esterase inhibitor and C4 are decreased.
    c) Typically, swelling lasts 3-5 days.
    d) May be an acquired disorder in lymphoproliferative disease or carcinoma

For the following set of questions, assign each feature to the correct autoimmune bullous disease.

A. Bullous pemphigoid
B. Pemphigus vulgarus
C. Dermatitis herpetiformis

52. Associated with disease that is in turn associated with anti-reticulin antibody
53. Flaccid bullae
54. Granular deposits of IgA in the dermal papillae
55. IgG vs. the basement membrane
56. Intensely pruritic, chronic papulovesicular skin disease characterized by lesions symmetrically distributed over extensor surfaces
57. Intraepidermal disease
58. Responsive to dapsone and a gluten-free diet
59. Management generally requires the most immunosuppressive.
60. Titre of IgG correlates to disease activity.

For the following set of questions, match each description with the appropriate diagnosis on fingernail examination.

A. Telangiectasia plus nailfold infarcts
B. Half-and-half (Terry's) nails
C. Koilonychia (spoon nails)
D. Onycholysis
E. Müehrckles lines
F. Mee's lines
G. Beau's lines

61. Arsenic poisoning
62. CHF and low albumin cirrhosis
63. Chronic iron deficiency
64. Collagen vascular disease
65. Hypoalbuminemia associated with nephrotic syndrome
66. Temporary arrest of nail plate function following disease or chemotherapy
67. Thyrotoxicosis, onychomycosis, psoriasis may cause

For the next set of questions match each description with the associated type of erythema.

A. Erythema Nodosum
B. Erythema Chronicum Migrans
C. Erythema Marginatum
D. Erythema Multiforme
E. Erythema Gyratum Repens
F. Necrolytic Migratory Erythema

68. Breast Carcinoma

69. Glucagonoma

70. Lyme Disease

71. Rheumatic Fever

72. Sarcoidosis

73. Stevens-Johnson Syndrome

74. Each of the following has a known association with erythema nodosum except:

a) Lofgren's syndrome
b) Behçet's disease
c) Ulcerative colitis
d) Henoch-Schönlein syndrome

75. Each of the following is considered a type of acanthosis nigricans except:

a) Vasculitis-associated AN
b) Hereditary benign AN
c) Pseudo AN
d) Drug-induced AN
e) Malignant AN

76. All of the following are true for Cutaneous T-cell Lymphoma (mycosis fungoides) except:

a) Lymph node and internal organ involvement are frequently seen.
b) This is a malignancy of suppressor (CD8+) T-cells.
c) Median length of survival is 5 years from the time of histological diagnosis.
d) The male: female ratio in this disorder is 27:1

77. A 55 yo man was recently diagnosed by his dermatologist with Sezary syndrome. All of the following are true about this disorder except:
    a) Sezary syndrome is a special variant of cutaneous T-cell lymphoma,
    b) It is characterized by generalized erythroderma, generalized LN, and cellular infiltrates of atypical lymphocytes (Sezary cells) in the skin and the blood.
    c) Erythroderma implies generalized redness of the skin along with a velvety, hyperpigmented rash.
    d) Buffy coat classically contains 15-30% atypical lymphocytes, but may be normal.
    e) Palms and soles commonly show diffuse hyperkeratosis.

78. An 18 yo female was recently diagnosed with tinea versicolor. All of the following are true about this disorder except:
    a) It is a chronic, asymptomatic scaling dermatosis associated with pityrosporum ovale, and is characterized by well-demarcated scaling macules with variable pigmentation, occurring most commonly on the trunk.
    b) Gentle abrasion of the surface accentuates the scaling.
    c) Low levels of cortisol increase susceptibility (e.g. congenital adrenal insufficiency).
    d) Humidity predisposes (increased incidence in summer time).

79. A 43 yo patient of yours with a known history of SLE presents with palpable purpura on her exam. The dermatologist tells you that SLE can cause a hypersensitivity vasculitis that presents in this way. All of the following are additional causes of hypersensitivity vasculitis except:
    a) Serum sickness
    b) Medications (e.g. isotretinoin and chlorpropamide)
    c) Hep B and C
    d) Essential mixed cryoglobulinemia
    e) Sjögren's syndrome

80. All of the following are correctly matched pairs of associations except:
    a) Hairy cell leukemia and polyarteritis nodosa (PAN)
    b) PAN and hepatitis B
    c) Cryoglobulinemia and hepatitis C
    d) Paroxysmal nocturnal hemoglobinuria and parvovirus B-19

81. A 27 yo HIV + man presents with 2 discrete, solid, skin-colored papules on his chest and 3 similar lesions on his face. The papules show central umbilication. What is the most likely diagnosis ?
    a) Cryptococcus neoformans
    b) Histoplasmosis
    c) Molluscum contagiosum
    d) Simple warts

For the following set of questions regarding Neurofibromatosis (NF), choose the form of disease (NF1 or NF2) that bears the features listed.

A. NF-1
B. NF-2
C. Both NF-1 and NF-2
D. Neither

82. Café-au-lait spots
83. Chromosome 17
84. Chromosome 22
85. Considered the "classic type"
86. Gliomas
87. Lisch nodules (pigmented hamartomas of the iris)
88. More common of the two
89. Multiple sclerosis
90. Pheochromocytoma
91. Unilateral acoustic neuromas

92. A 34 yo caucasian male presents to you with several large hyperpigmented lesions on his back. You diagnose these as dysplastic melanocytic nevi. All of the following accurately describe these lesions except:
    a) Acquired, circumscribed, pigmented lesions representing disordered proliferations of atypical melanocytes
    b) Autosomal dominant and more common in lighter skin races and may arise de novo or as part of a compound melanocytic nevus
    c) Considered potential precursors of superficial spreading melanoma and markers for persons at risk for developing primary malignant melanoma of the skin.
    d) Unlike common acquired nevi, new lesions are usually not seen after middle age.

93 All of the following accurately describe dermatologic manifestations of glucagonoma syndrome except:
    a) A superficial migratory necrolytic erythema with erosions that crust and heal with hyperpigmentation is often seen.
    b) This rash typically involves the central 1/3 face, groin, perineum & lower abdomen as well as extensor and frictional areas with blistering/hyperpigmentation
    c) The rash resolves or improves after tumor excision and is poorly responsive to medical treatment.
    d) Patients also commonly display a sore red tongue and angular cheilitis.

94. A 52 yo patient presents with new flat-topped violaceous papules over his knuckles, violaceous inflammatory changes over the eyelids and periorbital area, and increasing difficulty rising from his chair and walking up stairs. All of the following are true for patients with this disease except:

  a) Patients frequently display photosensitivity.
  b) Elevated CPK and aldolase are common.
  c) There is an association with interstitial pneumonitis and a five- to seven-fold increase in malignancies, especially testicular, hepatic, and hematologic.
  d) Poikiloderma is commonly noted in these individuals.

95. All of the following are true regarding the dermatologic manifestations of primary systemic amyloidosis except:

  a) "Pinch purpura" of the upper eyelid can appear as hemorrhagic papules after pinching or rubbing the eyelid.
  b) Scleroderma-like changes are seen in primary amyloidosis, and not in myeloma-associated amyloidosis, and are a useful way to differentiate the two.
  c) Patchy alopecia is a frequent dermatologic manifestation.
  d) Type AL is primary; AA is secondary. Usually there are no dermatologic findings in secondary type.

96. Icthyosis vulgaris, a generalized hyperkeratosis with xerosis producing rhomboidal fish-like scales most pronounced on the lower extremities, is associated with all of the following diseases except:

  a) Hodgkin's disease
  b) Intrinsic asthma
  c) Lung, breast, and cervical carcinomas
  d) Hypothyroidism
  e) AIDS

97. Each of the following is a characteristic feature of Sweet's syndrome except:

  a) Associated with ALL and lower respiratory infections
  b) Tender, red plaques predominantly distributed on the face, trunk, and extremities
  c) Also known as acute febrile neutrophilic dermatosis; arthralgia is frequently seen in this disease
  d) Prompt response to glucocorticoids.

98. A 68 yo male presents with weakness, weight loss, dysphagia, and a 2 week history of superficial blisters on non-inflamed skin over the past week. Rupture of several of these lesions has lead to large erosions. While he didn't mention it to his doctor until now, he also describes an additional 6 month history of painful oral lesions. A biopsy of one of the skin lesions reveals an intraepidermal blister and serum turned up antibody to intercellular substance. All of the following are true for this disease except:

a) The disease is increased in patients of Jewish descent.
b) Oral lesions are usually seen in 80-90% of all patients.
c) There is an association with myasthenia gravis and thymoma, and there is an increased incidence of lymphoreticular malignancy.
d) Nikolsky sign (i.e. application of pressure to an apparently uninvolved part of the skin triggers new bullae formation in 1-2 days) is highly characteristic.

99. A 48 yo female presents with a bullous eruption. On exam the bullae are tense and intact. Biopsy reveals that the bullae are subepidermal. The pathologist diagnoses bullous pemphigoid. All of the following are true for her disease except:

a) In contrast to pemphigus vulgaris, which can be acute or chronic, pemphigoid is chronic only.
b) The average age range of patients is 60-80 yo vs. 40-60 yo for pemphigus.
c) Circulating anti-basement membrane antibodies are seen in 70% of pemphigoid cases.
d) There is an association with breast, lung, and ovarian carcinoma in pemphigoid.

100. All of the following are true relating to sarcoidosis-associated diseases or syndromes except:

a) Lupus pernio is a particular type of sarcoidosis that involves the tip of the nose, cheeks, lips, ears, fingers, and knees, with lesions that are violaceous in color. This form of sarcoidosis is associated with involvement of the upper respiratory tract and is also seen in systemic lupus.
b) Löfgren's syndrome usually refers to the combination of E. nodosum + fever + arthralgias + bilateral hilar LN seen in a minority of acute presentations of sarcoidosis.
c) The Heerfordt syndrome represents a variety of sarcoidosis known as uveoparotid fever, in which patients manifest with fever, parotid enlargement, anterior uveitis, and facial nerve palsy.
d) When the lacrimal gland is involved, a keratoconjunctivitis sicca syndrome, with dry, sore eyes, can result.

101. Pseudoxanthoma elasticum bears all of the following associations except:

a) Mitral valve prolapse
b) Angioid streaks on the skin
c) Ischemic cardiac disease and peripheral vascular disease
d) GI hemorrhage

102. All of the following are features of dermatitis herpetiformis except:

a) Chronic, recurrent, intensely pruritic vesicles, papules, or urticarial wheals
b) Symmetric extensor surfaces, elbows, knees, scapula, buttocks
c) Nearly always associated with gluten-sensitive enteropathy
d) Granular IgG immunofluorescence pattern of infiltration in the skin

103. A 24 yo female presents with complaints of chronic, recurrent epistaxis requiring multiple visits to the E.R. and recently 2 episodes of hematochezia. Her father and paternal grandmother had also had a history of nose bleeds. On examination of the patient's lips and nasal mucosa, a number of telangiectasias are apparent. Colonoscopy later reveals the same findings in her colon. All of the following are true for her disease except:

a) This is an autosomal dominant disease
b) Treatment involves destruction of telangiectatic vessels using electrocautery or laser surgery with pulse dye laser.
c) Abnormal platelet function is also common.
d) Hemoptysis is usually secondary to pulmonary arteriovenous malformations (AVMs).

104. All of the following are true regarding Acrodermatitis Enteropathica except:

a) AE is an autosomal recessive disorder of Zn absorption.
b) This disease is apparently caused by an inborn error of metabolism resulting in malabsorption of dietary zinc and can be effectively treated only through parenteral administration of zinc.
c) The triad of AE includes acral dermatitis (face, hands, feet, anogenital area), alopecia, and diarrhea. The syndrome of acrodermatitis enteropathica includes severe desquamating skin lesions, intractable diarrhea, bizarre neurologic symptoms, variable combined immunodeficiency, and an often fatal outcome.
d) It is nearly identical clinically with acquired Zn deficiency due either to dietary deficiency or other absorptive disorder.

105. A patient presents with a history of an erythematous expanding annular rash with a central zone of clearing one week following a hunting trip in Connecticut. He reports no history of a tick bite. His only complaints are fatigue, malaise, headache, stiff neck, and myalgias. All of the following are true about this disease except:

a) Average duration of the rash is usually 3 weeks.
b) Only 14% of patients report a history of a tick bite.
c) Removal of the tick within 8 hours may preclude infection.
d) Long-term complication, if untreated, may include arthritis, myo/pericarditis, and cranial nerve palsies.

106. Which of the following statements is true regarding scleroderma?

a) It is generally classified as limited (40%) or diffuse (60%) scleroderma.
b) Patients with limited form usually have a long history of Raynaud's phenomenon.
c) Limited scleroderma manifests Scl-70 autoantibody in a majority of cases.
d) Anticentromere antibody is common in diffuse scleroderma.

107. All of the following are true statements regarding morphea except:

a) Male to female ratio is approximately 3:1
b) The lesion manifests as an indurated, poorly defined plaque with a central yellow so-called "carnauba wax"-colored area surrounded by a lilac border.
c) It is also known as "localized scleroderma", "circumscribed scleroderma".
d) In some patients, borrelia burgdorferi may be the causative agent.

108. True statements about GVHD (graft versus host disease) include all of the following except:

a) GVHD is an immune disorder seen primarily in allogeneic bone marrow transplants .
b) The acute form is usually seen between 14-21 days post-transplant.
c) The chronic form is seen >30 days post-transplant; may arise 2° to acute *or* de novo.
d) Chronic manifestations may include: lichenoid eruptions and sclerodermatous changes; wasting; chronic liver disease; skin/joint contractures; permanent hair loss; and xerostomia/xeropthalmia.

109. Each of the following is true concerning measles except:

a) Koplik's spots (cluster of tiny bright red papules on the throat appearing on or after the 2nd day of febrile illness) are pathognomonic.
b) Spread is generally from the face and neck to the trunk and extremities in 2-3 days.
c) Spread occurs via respiratory droplet aerosols (sneezing, coughing).
d) A hacking, bark-like cough is common.

110. A 42 yo male presents to you in early August after having just returned from a vacation through Costa Rica, Panama, Columbia, and Brazil. He complains of a several-day history of fever, chills, severe headache, and photophobia prior to the onset of a rash. His wife, with whom he traveled, describes the lesions began 2 days ago before flying back to the states, and after several days of fever, chills, and headache. Initially they were red on his wrists, ankles, palms, and soles. As you examine him, you now notice lesions have spread to his trunk, and are, for the most part erythematous macules and papules; some, however, are purpuric. All of the following are true for this patient's disease except:

a) Generally, the pattern of spread of disease is considered to be "centripetal".
b) The disease is relatively rare in the Rocky Mountain states.
c) Dermacentor andersonii accounts for most of the cases in the Western United States.
d) Patients may present with diffuse vasculitis, hypernatremia, and reactive thrombocytosis.

111. All of the following are true regarding ecthyma gangrenosum except:

a) Pseudomonas aeruginosa is the causative agent.
b) It is considered a necrotizing cellulitis.
c) Usually multiple lesions are seen.
d) Most commonly seen in the setting of profound and/or prolonged neutropenia

112. A 52 yo female presents with a painful facial cellulitis with a raised margin that is sharply demarcated from surrounding normal tissue. All of the following are likely to be true for this disease except:

a) It is usually caused by group A streptococcus.
b) It is a relatively rare cause of virulent soft tissue infection in a healthy host.
c) It is a superficial type of cellulitis involving lymphatics.
d) Sites of predilection include face; lower legs; and areas of preexisting lymphedema.

113. A fisherman presents to you with a severe, painful cellulitis of his right hand. He describes that his whole family are fish-handlers. On exam you note a painful, swollen purplish-red lesion with a sharply defined irregular raised border. All of the following are true regarding this patient's disease except:

a) An acute and rapidly evolving cellulitis occurring at sites of inoculation, most commonly the hands, is typical.
b) It is associated with occupational exposure, especially handling fish, shellfish, meat, poultry, hides, and bones.
c) Erysipelothrix rhusiopathiae, a gram-positive rod is the causative agent.
d) Treatment is either penicillin or erythromycin.

114. All of the following are true statements regarding scarlet fever except:

a) One of the dermatologic signs is so-called Pastia's lines, which describes erythema in skin folds such as neck, axillae, groin, antecubital and popliteal fossae.
b) Group A Streptococcus is the culprit organism accounting for the pharyngitis, accompanied by a characteristic rash. The rash arises from the effects of one of three toxins, which are currently designated streptococcal pyrogenic exotoxins A, B, and C.
c) The rash appears within 1-3 days of infection and erythema is first noted on the trunk and spreads to the extremities. Palms and soles are usually always involved.
d) The exanthem fades within 4-5 days and is followed by brawny desquamation on the body and extremities and by sheet-like exfoliation on the palms and soles.

115. All of the following are true for cat scratch fever except:

a) Bartonella henselae (formerly Rochmalimaea henselae) is the causative organism, which in HIV-infected patients causes bacillary angiomatosis.
b) Nodes are usually solitary, moderately tender, and freely mobile. They are suppurative, and the white blood cell count is usually normal.
c) CSD is a serious zoonotic infection. IV erythromycin is the treatment of choice in most cases.
d) Warthin-Starry-stained sections of skin lesion , conjunctiva, or lymph nodes show small, pleomorphic bacilli. Antibodies to B. henselae are usually pos (>= 1:64); PCR is 96% sensitive from aspirations of infected lymph nodes.

116. A 29 yo female presents with complaints of years of "acne", for which she has never sought treatment. She also describes pronounced facial flushing in response to heat, emotional stimuli, alcohol, hot drinks, and spicy foods that seems to be getting worse over the past month. On exam you find papules, pustules, and telangiectasias in her malar regions. All of the following are true about her disease except:

a) The disease is seen more commonly in women. The most severe cases are usually in men.
b) Long standing may lead to connective tissue overgrowth, particularly of the nose (rhinophyma).
c) It is often differentiated from acne vulgaris by its lack of comedones and the characteristic history.
d) It is more common in those of northern European descent.

117. A 45 yo Japanese male presents with complaints of recurrent canker sores, "red eyes", and painful, red nodules on his arms and legs. All of the following are additional features of his disease except:

a) Most recent diagnostic criteria include one basic major feature--recurrent oral apthous ulcers--and 2 of the following features: recurrent genital apthous ulcers; eye lesions (posterior uveitis); skin lesions (E. nodosum-like lesions, or cutaneous pustular vasculitis)
b) Spontaneous thrombophlebitis
c) Positive pathergy test: placement of an anergy panel to at least 2 fungal antigens (e.g. candida and trichophyton) reveals no response at 24-48 hours.
d) The patient is likely to be HLA B5 with a seronegative arthritis.

118. An AIDS patient presents with new macular rash to his lower extremities that is soon diagnosed as Kaposi's Sarcoma. All of the following are true regarding this disease except:

a) Linked to HHV-8, or human herpes virus type 8
b) Almost all KS lesions are palpable, even macules.
c) CDC case definition is that in a patient <60 yo, KS is an AIDS-defining condition if the patient has no other cause of immunodeficiency and is without knowledge of HIV Ab status.
d) Pulmonary and GI involvement in KS will usually be symptomatic.

119. A 57 yo female 40 pack-year smoker presents with a "white rash" on her buccal mucosa that she had noticed while brushing her teeth. Examination reveals a sharply defined, white, macular-to-slightly raised area on her left buccal mucosa. The whitish rash could not be rubbed off. All of the following are true regarding the most likely diagnosis in this patient except:

a) Candida albicans may secondarily invade.
b) It is considered a premalignant lesion since it is caused by exposure to the same agents that cause squamous cell ca: smoking, alcohol, chronic irritation/inflammation, HPV-11 and HPV-16.
c) About 10% of lesions can progress to malignancy. Buccal involvement is serious, with over 60% showing either carcinoma in situ or invasive SCC whereas lesions on the floor of the mouth are almost always benign.
d) Careful follow-up is important with biopsies to r/o dyplasia or frank carcinoma.

120. A patient presented to his physician with a chronic rash that turned out to be urticarial vasculitis. All of the following are true regarding this disorder except:

a) It is a multisystem disease with cutaneous lesions resembling urticaria, typically lasting <24 hours.
b) Leukocytoclastic vasculitis is seen with fever, arthralgias, increased ESR
c) May be seen in serum sickness; collagen vascular diseases; and HepB
d) Hypocomplementemia is seen 70% of the time.

121. All of the following correctly describe Beau's lines except:

a) Beau's lines are the horizontal depressions across the nail plate that are caused by a transient arrest in nail growth.
b) They may appear as white lines, when caused by arsenic.
c) It is possible to estimate the date of illness by the distance of the furrow from the proximal nail fold. As a rule of thumb, in an average patient, the nail plate takes 3-4 months to grow from its base to the distal edge.
d) Beau's lines may be seen in high fever, shock, MI, and pulmonary embolus.

122. A 33 yo male alcoholic presents with periorbital and malar violaceous coloration, hyperpigmentation, and hypertrichosis on the face in addition to bullae, crust, and scars on the dorsa of his hands. He is diagnosed with porphyria cutanea tarda (PCT). All of the following are true for PCT except:

a) Patients usually present with photosensitivity and complaints of "fragile skin", vesicles, and bullae, particularly on the dorsum of the hands, esp. after minor trauma.
b) The diagnosis is confirmed by the presence of an orange-red fluorescence of the urine under Wood's lamp.
c) Unlike variegate and intermittent acute porphyrias, PCT lacks acute, life-threatening attacks (abdominal pain, peripheral autonomic neuropathy, and respiratory failure)
d) Most PCT are induced by drugs (especially ethanol and estrogens) and are not hereditary.

123. All of the following are true regarding porphyria cutanea tarda except:

a) Diabetes, Hep C, and AIDS can predispose to PCT.
b) Increased plasma and hepatic iron are usually present.
c) Important in differentiating variegate porphyria (besides the lack of acute symptoms) is to check the stool for protoporphyrins (+ in PCT, - in VP).
d) Treatment includes discontinuation of offending agents; phlebotomy (qw or qow to Hgb <10) + low-dose chloroquine.

124. All of the following are true regarding pseudoporphyria and its relationship to porphyria cutanea tarda (PCT) except:

a) Pseudoporphyria is a vesiculobullous cutaneous condition that clinically and histologically resembles several of the features of porphyria cutanea tarda.
b) Pseudoporphyria displays several of the same biochemical porphyrin abnormalities as PCT.
c) Enhanced skin fragility and bullae formation on sun-exposed skin surfaces are the prominent features of pseudoporphyria.
d) In contrast to PCT, the presence of milia, hypertrichosis, alteration of pigmentation, sclerodermatous changes, and photo-onycholysis is generally lacking. Lesions are usually asymptomatic.

125. The differential diagnosis of essential mixed cryoglobulinemia includes all of the following except:
a) Raynaud's phenomenon
b) Hepatitis B and C
c) Livedo reticularis
d) Henoch-Schönlein Purpura

126. In addition to inflammatory bowel disease, pyoderma gangrenosum is associated with each of the following diseases except:
   a) Behçet's disease
   b) Multiple myeloma
   c) Leukemia
   d) Myelofibrosis

1. All of the following statements are true regarding Meniere's disease except:
    a) The classic triad is vertigo, tinnitus, and hearing loss.
    b) You need not have the entire triad present to make the diagnosis, but you must have the vertigo.
    c) 30% of cases of Meniere's disease are bilateral.
    d) The hearing loss is progressive and conductive.

2. All of the following statements are true regarding Myasthenia Gravis except:
    a) MG is often heralded by cranial nerve findings such as diplopia and dysarthria.
    b) Eaton-Lambert Syndrome is an important differential. It can be distinguished from MG since ELS patients derive *increased* strength from repeated activity, while MG patients get *weaker*.
    c) Eaton-Lambert syndrome is a paraneoplastic manifestation of oat cell carcinoma.
    d) Physostigmine or pyridostigmine are used in treating MG.
    e) The association of MG and thymoma is well known. Among patients with thymoma, approximately 30% go onto develop MG.

3. All of the following statements are true regarding Guillain Barre Syndrome except:
    a) Half the patients have a mild respiratory or GI infection 1-3 weeks prior to the onset of their GBS.
    b) GBS manifests as a severe, rapidly progressive, symmetric polyneuropathy that starts in the upper extremities and descends with pronounced proximal muscle weakness
    c) Weakness in the diaphragmatic muscles accounts for the respiratory weakness that can lead to ventilatory support.
    d) It is important to monitor GBS patients with Negative Inspiratory Pressures and Vital Capacities. If serial Negative Inspiratory Pressures are noted to become more positive, ventilatory support should be instituted prophylactically.

4. Emergent indications for the use of MRI include all of the following except:
    a) Patient has a history of breast carcinoma and now presents with lower extremity weakness.
    b) Patient presents with percussion tenderness over the spine.
    c) A patient taking prednisone 10 mg for the past 10 years for his polymyalgia rheumatica now presents with hip pain.
    d) Patient presents with lower back pain for the past 6 months now complaining of tingling, numbness, and dysesthesias along her lower extremity in the dermatomal distribution of L2.
    e) Patient presents with pain in her lower back worse with walking downstairs, but better on spinal flexion.

5. All of the following statements are true regarding Meralgia Paresthetica except:
   a) It is seen mostly in diabetics and is accompanied by paresthesias, weakness, atrophy, and pain in the thigh muscles.
   b) It results from compression to the lateral cutaneous nerve as it passes through the inguinal ligament.
   c) It can present with numbness or burning sensation over the outside of the thigh
   d) Prolonged standing or walking can promote symptoms.
   e) While weight loss may help, generally, it *spontaneously* subsides.

6. All of the following statements are true regarding seizures except:
   a) Head trauma is the chief cause of focal seizures in young adults, as opposed to brain tumor and vascular disease in older patients.
   b) Seizure disorder is an EEG and not a "clinical" diagnosis.
   c) Valproic acid is associated with neural tube defects.
   d) Three anticonvulsant that *reduce* the levels of oral contraceptive medications include dilantin, carbamazepine, and phenobarbital.
   e) Regarding anticonvulsant blood levels, therapeutic levels represent only average bell-shaped curves and should not be changed based on blood levels alone

7. All of the following statements are true regarding Pseudotumor Cerebri except:
   a) High opening pressures have been noted in animal studies.
   b) Mental status changes is a common of pseudotumor cerebri.
   c) If papilledema is noted, lumbar puncture should not be performed, *even if* the CT is negative for intracranial mass.
   d) Papilledema may be seen on fundoscopic examination. Enlarging blind spots and loss of peripheral vision are additional opthalmic features.
   e) Most patients are young, female, and obese.

8. All of the following are considered minor risk factors in cardioembolic sources of ischemic stroke except:
   a) Patent foramen ovale
   b) LV regional wall abnormalities
   c) Severe mitral annular calcification
   d) MVP
   e) Mitral stenosis

9. All of the following are true statements about subarachnoid hemorrhage except:
   a) SAH commonly presents with meningismus.
   b) SAH may present with a partial 3rd nerve or a 6th nerve palsy.
   c) The cranial nerve palsies seen in SAH are 2° to aneurysmal expansion.
   d) Most cases patients will have a warning or "sentinel" headache.
   e) Vomiting is a common feature of SAH.

For questions # 10-18 match all the fundoscopic findings to the appropriate disease. Answer either A or B.

A. Hypertension
B. Diabetes mellitus

10. 'Dot and blot' hemorrhages
11. Arterial-venous nicking
12. Flame hemorrhages
13. Hard exudates
14. Microaneurysms
15. Neovascularization
16. Papilledema
17. Silver/copper wiring
18. Soft exudates

19. All of the following are true statements about Ramsay-Hunt syndrome except:
    a) It is caused by herpes simplex virus to the geniculate ganglion of cranial nerve seven.
    b) Physical examination often reveals herpetic vesicles in the external ear.
    c) Patients may present with vertigo, nystagmus, and deafness.
    d) It should be included in the differential diagnosis of facial paralysis.

Question # 20-25 are matching-type questions. Three facial pain syndromes are listed. Match each feature with one of these syndromes.

A. Trigeminal neuralgia
B. Intracavernous internal carotid artery aneurysm
C. Post-herpetic neuralgia

20. Generally seen in patients > 50yo
21. May lead to opthalmoplegia, esp CN III
22. Most common among the elderly
23. Pain in the opthalmic branch of CN V
24. Sensory loss/pain to the opthalmic $\pm$ maxillary branches of CN V
25. The pain commonly involves the maxillary and mandibular branches of the 5th cranial nerve

For the following set of questions on hearing loss examination using the Weber and Rinne tests, choose the one best answer.

A. Conduction deafness
B. Nerve deafness

26. Lateralizes to deaf side on Weber's test
27. Bone conduction > Air conduction on the affected side on Rinne's test
28. Lateralizes to normal side on Weber's test
29. Air conduction > Bone conduction on both sides on Rinne's test

30. All of the following are important in the determination of brain death except:

    a) Absent gag/corneal/cough reflexes
    b) Loss of oculovestibular and oculocephalic reflexes
    c) No response to painful stimuli, except for spinal reflexes
    d) EEG if brain stem reflexes are persistently absent.

For the next set of questions match each interpretive EEG pattern with the correct diagnosis.

A. Myasthenia gravis
B. Eaton-Lambert syndrome
C. Myotonia
D. Polymyositis

31. 'Dive-bomber' reflexes (high frequency action potentials)
32. Decremental response to tetanic stimulation
33. Fibrillation (brief low-amplitude action potentials due to denervation hypersensitivity at the motor end plate)
34. Incremental response to repetitive stimulation

35. All of the following conditions are known risk factors for the development of cerebral aneurysms except:

    a) Polycystic kidney disease
    b) Ehlers-Danlos syndrome
    c) Renal artery stenosis due to fibromuscular dysplasia
    d) Aortic stenosis

36. All of the following conditions are true statements regarding management of Parkinson's disease except:
    a) Drug therapy should be initiated only when symptoms have a negative impact on the patient's ability to function.
    b) Levodopa (L-Dopa) is the most effective drug for PD; it is used in combination with carbidopa.
    c) A patient's failure to respond to one dopamine antagonist is usually a sign that s/he will not respond to another.
    d) Tolcapone, one of the newer agents, inhibits dopa metabolism in plasma and allows higher amounts of L-Dopa to cross the blood-brain barrier without increasing the L-Dopa dose.

For the next set of question match each description with the type of vertigo it describes.

A. Vestibular
B. Benign Positional Vertigo
C. Labyrinthitis
D. Vestibular ototoxicity

37. A vertigo brought about by specific head positions such as while rolling over in bed or arising from bed in the morning.

38. Felt to be 2° to viral infection to the vestibular nerve/ vestibular apparatus and usually lasts a few weeks.

39. May be the result of bacterial or viral infection.

40. Usually a more chronic condition, accompanied by disequilibrium and hearing loss.

41. A 55 yo male with a known history of an extrapyramidal syndrome presents with repeated falls accompanied by nuchal dystonia and paralysis of voluntary downgaze. All of the following are true about this disorder except:

    a) It is a sporadic degenerative disorder characterized pathologically by neuronal loss, gliosis, and neurofibrillary tangles in the midbrain, pons, basal ganglia, and dentate nuclei of the cerebellum.
    b) There is conspicuous failure of voluntary saccadic gaze in a vertical plane, especially downward, with later involvement of horizontal gaze. Eventually, smooth pursuit movements are also affected.
    c) Axial dystonia in extension, especially of the neck, is common and is frequently accompanied by limb rigidity and bradykinesia that may mimic Parkinson's disease.
    d) Resting tremor is another common feature that can look like Parkinson's disease.

For the next set of questions match each characteristic with the appropriate type of tremor it describes.

A. Essential
B. Parkinsonian
C. Cerebellar

42. Tremor is best seen with certain postures
43. Tremor is best seen at rest
44. Aggravated by action
45. Aggravated by stress/anxiety
46. Relieved by rest
47. Relieved by alcohol
48. Associated features include voice, head, and chin tremors
49. Most common etiology is familial.

50. A 35 yo female presents with weakness in her limbs, "pins and needles" sensation in her right forearm, ataxia, trouble recalling things she used to have no problem remembering, and decreasing attention span. Additionally, exam reveals loss of dexterity, hyperreflexia, and a mild dysarthria. You decide to order an MRI to confirm your suspicion, and expect to see periventricular white matter ischemia, which you do. All of the following are true regarding the most likely diagnosis except:

    a) Patients frequently note increased exacerbations in cold weather.
    b) Depression and labile mood are common psychiatric concomitants.
    c) Optic neuritis is a common manifestation.
    d) Oligoclonal bands may be seen on examination of the cerebrospinal fluid.

For the next set of questions match each prodromal clinical descriptor with its actual meaning as related to migraine with aura.

A. Fortification spectra
B. Photopsia
C. Scotomata
D. Teichopsia

51. "Blind spots"
52. Bright shimmering or wavy lines
53. Flashing lights
54. Zigzag pattern resembling the facade of a physical structure

For the following set of questions match each disorder with the correct abnormal pupil size on exam.

A. Small pupils
B. Large pupils

55. Amphetamine overdose
56. Argyll Robertson pupil
57. Atropine poisoning
58. Holmes-Adie pupil
59. Horner's syndrome
60. Opiates
61. Pilocarpine drops
62. Pontine bleed

For the following set of questions, match each disorder to the type of tremor that may be associated.

A. At rest tremor
B. Intention tremor

63. Anxiety, alcohol
64. Benign essential tremor, mild
65. Cerebellar disease
66. Multiple sclerosis
67. Severe Parkinsonism
68. Stroke
69. Thyrotoxicosis
70. Wilson's tremor

71. Each of the following is considered a poor prognostic sign in Bell's palsy except:
    a) Trismus
    b) Paralysis of stapedius muscle
    c) Severe taste impairment
    d) Reduced lacrimation

72. All of the following conditions have known associations with Restless Legs Syndrome except:
    a) Rheumatoid arthritis
    b) Pregnancy
    c) Smoking
    d) Peripheral neuropathy
    e) Iron and folate deficiencies

GERIATRICS

For questions # 1-6, match the clinical finding with the appropriate type of urinary incontinence.

A. Stress incontinence
B. Urge incontinence
C. Overflow incontinence

1. Abnormal bladder contractions/detrusor instability are responsible
2. Association with estrogen deficient states
3. Bladder overdistension is responsible
4. BPH, fecal impaction may induce
5. Small amounts of leaking with such activities as sneezing, laughing, coughing, jumping
6. Urethral hypermobility/internal sphinctor deficiency responsible

7. Each of the following labs is noted to increase with age except:
   a) Uric acid
   b) Alkaline phosphatase
   c) Triglycerides
   d) WBC
   e) Fasting blood glucose

8. Each of the following labs is noted to decrease with age except:
   a) Serum albumin
   b) HDL
   c) CPK
   d) Creatinine clearance
   e) TSH

9. All of the following statements are true with regards to sleep patterns in aging except:
   a) There is no change in sleep requirements.
   b) There is an ↑ in nocturnal awakenings.
   c) There is a ↓ in sleep latency.
   d) There is a ↓ in both REM *and* deep sleep.
   e) There is decreased sleep efficiency.

10. All of the following are true statements regarding subcortical dementias except:
    a) Subcortical dementia is manifest in Alzheimer's disease.
    b) Parkinson's disease and multi-infarct dementia are examples.
    c) Subcortical dementias are characterized by prominent motor abnormalities and by changes in mood, personality, and difficulty with planning.
    d) Changes in impulse control may be seen.

ALLERGY & IMMUNOLOGY QUESTIONS

1. Treatment of the acute symptoms of anaphylaxis includes all of the following except:
   a) Antihistamines
   b) Epinephrine
   c) Fluids
   d) Steroids
   e) Oxygen

2. True statements about anaphylactoid reactions include all of the following except:
   a) The main cause is radiocontrast media.
   b) They resemble anaphylactic reactions in most ways.
   c) They are mediated by IgE.
   d) Skin tests are not used in diagnosis.

3. Examples of causes of anaphylactoid reactions include all of the following except:
   a) Medications such as penicillin
   b) Dialysis
   c) Physical stimuli, like cold and exercise
   d) Plasma expanders
   e) Transfusion reactions

4. True statements about reactions to radiocontrast media include all of the following except:
   a) Reactions are 2° to high osmolality of contrast media.
   b) Lower osmolar media are better received.
   c) There is a correlation with shellfish allergy and iodine.
   d) If the patient has had a bad reaction in the past, s/he has a 20-35% risk of similar reaction on reexposure to these media.
   e) A combination of prednisone, diphenhydramine, and ephedrine can prevent approximately 90% of these reactions.

Questions # 5-12 are matching questions related to immune reaction types I-IV. Find the one best answer.

A. Type I
B. Type II
C. Type III
D. Type IV

5. Also known as the Arthrus reaction
6. Cytotoxic cells play a key role in the pathogenesis
7. Delayed hypersensitivity
8. Demonstrates a "wheal and flare" response

9. Examples include allergic rhinitis and asthmatic urticaria
10. Examples include Goodpasture's disease, Graves' disease, and immune hemolytic anemia
11. Examples include rheumatoid arthritis, SLE, and Hep B viral prodrome
12. Examples include the PPD test, contact dermatitis, and GVHD

13. True statements about RAST testing include all of the following except:
    a) Measure specific IgE to various antigens.
    b) RAST testing is less specific, but more sensitive than skin testing.
    c) RAST is indicated in those individuals who are so exquisitely sensitive to an antigen that skin testing may induce a systemic reaction.
    d) RAST is appropriate for patients who are unable to discontinue certain medications that would otherwise affect skin testing results.

Questions # 14-22 are matching questions on Immunodeficiency Diseases. Choose one best answer by matching appropriate clinical examples to the defects responsible.

A. B cells
B. T cells
C. Neutrophils
D. Terminal components
E. C3
F. C6,7
G. C1 esterase inhibitor

14. Chronic granulomatous disease; Chediak Higashi disease
15. Hereditary angioedema
16. Ig A deficiency
17. Pyogenic infections
18. Raynaud's phenomenon
19. Recurrent infections with extracellular, encapsulated bacteria
20. Recurrent neisseria infections
21. TB, fungal, toxoplasmosis infections
22. X-linked agammaglobulinemia

For the next set of questions assign each characteristic to either T cells or B cells.

A. T cells
B. B cells

23. Cell-mediated immunity against intercellular organisms
24. Majority are fixed and immobile; 20% circulate
25. Most are long-lived memory cells

For the following set match each idiopathic disease with the correct HLA (A,B, or C loci) that can be associated.

A. A3
B. B27
C. B35
D. Cw6
E. B5
F. B2, B9
G. B8

26. Acute anterior uveitis
27. Acute lymphocytic leukemia--associated with prolonged survival
28. Behçet's disease
29. de Quervain's subacute thyroiditis
30. Hemochromatosis
31. Hodgkin's disease-- associated with prolonged survival
32. Psoriasis

Now match the immunological disease to the HLA (usually DR) with which it is often associated.

A. DR2
B. DR3
C. DR4
D. DR5
E. DR3 *and* DR4

33. Anti-glomerular basement membrane disease
34. Celiac disease
35. Graves' disease
36. IDDM
37. Multiple sclerosis
38. Myasthenia gravis
39. Pernicious anemia
40. Rheumatoid arthritis
41. Sjögren's disease
42. SLE

43. Which of the following is *not* considered an indication for plasmapheresis in the subset of patients who do not respond to conventional treatment?
    a) ITP
    b) Goodpasture's syndrome
    c) Rapidly progressive glomerulonephritis
    d) Essential cryoglobulinemia
    e) Myasthenia gravis
    f) CLL

1. Causes of low voltage EKG include all of the following except:

   a) Cardiac tamponade
   b) Pectus excavatum
   c) Obesity
   d) Cardiomyopathy
   e) Pericardial effusion

2. Causes of Tall R-wave (R>S) in leads V1 or V2 include all of the following except:

   a) Posterior wall MI
   b) RBBB
   c) Left anterior fascicular block
   d) WPW
   e) Right axis deviation

3. Pathological Q-waves may be caused by all of the following except:

   a) Hyperkalemia
   b) LBBB
   c) Transmural MI
   d) Myocardial Ischemia
   e) WPW

4. The differential diagnosis of ↑ QTc interval includes all of the following except:

   a) Hypomagnesemia, hypocalcemia
   b) Pentamidine
   c) Thyrotoxicosis
   d) Tricyclic antidepressants
   e) Amiodarone

5. All of the following are true statements about posterior wall MI except:

   a) EKG shows tall, widened R and T waves in V1,V2
   b) Can see upsloping ST depression in V1,V2
   c) Usually associated with signs of inferior wall MI
   d) The main blood distribution to the posterior wall is the left anterior descending artery.
   e) Right-sided leads may be placed in order to flesh out a posterior wall MI.

6. All of the following are true statements about U-waves except:

    a) They are an important prognosticator post MI if seen in the first 2 days.
    b) They follow the T-wave and are inverted just like the letter "U"
    c) They may be a normal variant.
    d) Electrolyte imbalances are often responsible.

7. Each of the following statements are true about poor R-wave progression except:

    a) In general the height of the R-wave should increase as you move from the right side of the precordium to the left.
    b) Normally, one should see an R-wave height of 3mm by V3 or 4mm by V4.
    c) If the R-wave if V4>R-wave in V3, this is referred to as "regression" and is usually evidence of infarct expansion.
    d) Prolonged inspiration can masquerade as poor R-wave progression.

8. In order to make the diagnosis of right ventricular hypertrophy, all of the following must be ruled out except:

    a) RBBB
    b) Left posterior hemiblock
    c) Anterolateral or inferior wall MI
    d) S>R in V5, V6

9. All of the following are relative contraindications to the use of thrombolytic agents in the setting of an acute MI except:

    a) Surgery or trauma in the past 2 weeks
    b) CVA within the previous 6 months
    c) GI bleed within 1 month
    d) Pregnancy
    e) BP> 200/110

10. Which one of the following agents commonly causes hypotension as a side effect?

    a) APSAC
    b) Streptokinase
    c) TPA
    d) Urokinase

11. Which of the following statements is LEAST likely to be true?

a) Generally, for acute MI, one must have ST elevations of 1mm in the limb leads and 2mm in the V (chest) leads.
b) While there are definite size criteria for pathologic or significant Q-waves, any Q-wave, even 'baby' Q-waves, are significant if seen in V1 or V2.
c) Routine prophylactic use of lidocaine post MI should be avoided as it can increase mortality by causing ventricular tachycardia.
d) Treatment of posterior wall and right ventricular myocardial infarctions includes nitroprusside to assist in decreasing the myocardial wall stress.

12. In interpreting EKGs, which of the following statements is least likely to be true?

a) One cannot include a lateral component to an inferior wall MI if there are only T-wave inversions laterally. There must be either ST elevations or Q-waves.
b) For a posterior component to an inferior wall MI, it is best to look at V1 and V2 for R>S and/or ST↓ ≥ 2mm. If, however, there is a right bundle branch block with the inferior wall MI, right-sided leads should be checked to rule out a posterior component.
c) ST elevations are common in unstable angina; aspirin and heparin have been proved to decrease mortality in this condition.
d) Asymmetric T-waves are 'asymmetric' because they involve ST segment ↑, which is why they usually suggest acute MI or ischemia.

13. Digoxin toxicity can cause a multitude of arrhythmias. However, there are two that are considered the 'sine qua non' of digoxin toxicity. They are:

a) Mobitz I and atrial fibrillation
b) SA exit block and PAT with 2:1 block
c) Mobitz II and VTach
d) Sinus arrest and WPW

14. All of the following are correct statements regarding pacemaker syndrome except:

a) It is sometimes seen in patients with VVI pacemakers; dual chamber pacing is frequently corrective.
b) EKG typically reveals retrograde P-waves.
c) The pacemaker syndrome consists of fatigue, dizziness, syncope, and distressing pulsations in the neck and chest and can be associated with adverse hemodynamic effects.
d) Patients are usually short of breath on exertion, but relieved by rest.

15. All of the following are important criteria in diagnosing left anterior hemiblock except:
    a) QRS between .08-.10s
    b) Left axis deviation > -45°
    c) Small Q in inferior leads, and deep S in leads I and L
    d) Small R waves inferiorly

16. All of the following are true regarding complete heart block (CHB) and AV dissociation (AVD) except:
    a) When the atrial rate exceeds the ventricular rate, that is CHB.
    b) When the ventricular rate exceeds the atrial rate, that is AVD.
    c) Cannon "a" waves can occur in either CHB or AVD.
    d) Differentiating these two is important as the management differs.

For the next three questions, match each situation to the appropriate recommendation regarding atrial fibrillation and conversion to normal sinus rhythm.

A. May attempt to chemically convert without anticoagulation
B. Must give anticoagulation approximately 3 weeks before and 3 weeks after converting to normal sinus rhythm
C. The goal is to control ventricular response rate with meds such as digoxin, since it is less likely to convert

17. Atria < 5cm & atrial fibrillation > 2 days
18. Atria < 5cm & atrial fibrillation ≤ 2 days
19. Atria > 5cm & atrial fibrillation > 2 days

20. All of the following are true statements concerning cardiogenic shock except:
    a) Insertion of an intraaortic balloon pump decreases ventricular afterload, improving myocardial performance and decreasing myocardial oxygen demand and improving coronary perfusion pressure by increasing aortic diastolic pressure.
    b) The possibility of acute mechanical abnormalities such as mitral regurgitation or ventricular septal defect should be excluded, with either echocardiography or right heart catheterization.
    c) Where possible, it is probably best to perform emergent coronary angiography to define the coronary anatomy and to attempt revascularization.
    d) Cardiogenic shock can also occur after prolonged cardiopulmonary bypass; the hibernating myocardium may require hours or days to recover sufficiently to support the circulation.

21. All of the following are true concerning the intraaortic balloon pump (IABP) except:
    a) It works via decreasing ventricular afterload, improving myocardial performance and decreasing myocardial oxygen demand and improving coronary perfusion pressure by increasing aortic diastolic pressure.
    b) It is contraindicated in VSD, papillary muscle rupture, and refractory unstable angina.
    c) It is an important therapeutic modality in managing ventricular tachycardia 2° to ischemia.
    d) It can play a life-saving role in cardiogenic shock.

22. From the following choose the answer that is least likely to cause ventricular bigeminy:
    a) Digoxin toxicity
    b) Myxedema coma
    c) Acidemia or alkalemia
    d) Ischemia

23. Which of the following statements is least likely to be true regarding multifocal atrial tachycardia (MAT) ?
    a) Heart rate is usually > 105 bpm.
    b) At least 3 different P-wave morphologies should be seen.
    c) Verapamil and digoxin play a key role in the management of uncomplicated MAT.
    d) MAT is a complication of COPD.

24. All of the following are true regarding the diagnosis of wandering atrial pacemaker except:
    a) It can look like MAT since also usually see at least 3 P-wave morphologies.
    b) The rate in WAP is usually < 95, key in differentiating it from MAT.
    c) WAP is essentially ‘physiologic’, whereas MAT is considered ‘pathologic’.
    d) WAP is usually secondary to repositioning of the atrial lead in dual chamber pacemakers.

25. Which of the following interventions has *not* been shown to reduce mortality following myocardial infarction?
    a) Salicylates
    b) Nitrates
    c) ACE inhibitors
    d) Beta-blockers

26. All of the following are true regarding ASD except:

    a) It characteristically gives a widely split S2.
    b) Biatrial enlargement is common on the EKG.
    c) Pulmonary pressures are elevated.
    d) There are two types: secundum, which yields a *right* axis deviation and *does not* require endocarditis prophylaxis, and primum, which yields a *left* axis deviation and *does* require endocarditis prophylaxis.

For the next set of questions match the hemodynamics to the correct diagnosis.

A. Right ventricular infarction
B. Tamponade
C. Both A and B
D. Neither A nor B

27. Elevated right atrial pressures

28. Depressed pulmonary capillary wedge pressure

29. Depressed cardiac output

30. Each of the following is a clinical manifestation of cardiac tamponade except:
    a) Hypotension
    b) JVD
    c) Kussmaul's sign
    d) Pulsus alternans
    e) Distant heart sounds

31. All of the following medicines can increase the digoxin level, when coadministered, except:
    a) Quinidine
    b) Ciprofloxacin
    c) Verapamil
    d) Thiazides
    e) Amiodarone

32. All of the following are true regarding WPW except:
    a) Delta waves are characteristically seen.
    b) These patients often go into atrial fibrillation or flutter. Procainamide is used for rate control in these patients.
    c) The PR interval is short.
    d) WPW can manifest a "pseudoinfarction" pattern.
    e) Radiofrequency catheter ablation is the treatment of choice in patients who are asymptomatic; surgical ablation is recommended if symptomatic.

33. Of the following Goldman criteria, which is the most important risk factor or prognosticator:
   a) Atrial fibrillation
   b) Age >70
   c) Frequent PVCs
   d) Third heart sound

34. All of the following are true statements concerning the hemodynamics of pregnancy except:
   a) There is an increase in systemic vascular resistance
   b) There is an increase in blood volume
   c) There is an increase in cardiac output
   d) There is an increase in stroke volume

For questions # 35-42 match each of the classic complications given to the site of myocardial infarction with which it is more likely to be associated.

A. Anterior MI
B. Posterior MI

35. Associated RV infarction
36. Bradycardias; complete heart block
37. Free wall rupture; VSD
38. LV aneurysm
39. Mobitz I
40. Mobitz II
41. Papillary muscle dysfunction
42. Ventricular arrhythmias

For the next set of questions, choose the most appropriate recommendation to date for anticoagulation in nonvalvular atrial fibrillation based on age and risk factors for CVA.

A. Warfarin
B. Aspirin
C. Warfarin or aspirin
D. Neither

43. A 61 yo with risk factors
44. A 77 yo with no risk factors
45. A 70 yo with risk factors

46. A 64 yo with no risk factors
47. An 80 yo with risk factors
48. A 67 yo with no risk factors

For the next set of question match the type of pulse to the disorder in which it is seen.

A. Alternans
B. Bisferiens
C. Collapsing
D. Plateau and tardus
E. Paradoxus
F. Hyperkinetic
G. Dicrotic

49. Aortic insufficiency; patent ductus arteriosis
50. Mitral regurgitation and VSD
51. Aortic stenosis
52. Aortic insufficiency and hypertrophic cardiomyopathy
53. Dilated cardiomyopathy
54. Severe left ventricular dysfunction
55. Tamponade; constrictive pericarditis; asthma

For the next set of questions match each description or diagnosis with the correct hemodynamic finding.

A. a waves
B. v waves
C. x descent
D. y descent
E. Rapid 'y' descent
F. Slow/absent 'y' descent
G. Rapid 'x' descent
H. Fixed elevation
I. Absent hepatojugular reflux

56. Atrial relaxation
57. Common to constrictive pericarditis and tamponade
58. Common to constrictive pericarditis and tricuspid incompetence
59. Common to tamponade and tricuspid stenosis
60. Inferior vena cava obstruction or Budd-Chiari Syndrome
61. Normal tricuspid opening
62. Right atrial systole
63. Superior vena cava syndrome
64. Venous filling

65. Which of the following conditions is LEAST likely to yield a soft first heart sound ?

a) 1st degree AV block
b) Left ventricular failure
c) Mitral regurgitation
d) Mitral stenosis with a mobile valve

For the following set of questions match the type of split S2 to its most likely cause.

A. Fixed split
B. Loud A2
C. Narrow split with loud P2
D. Paradoxical
E. Physiologic
F. Single S2 (inaudible A2)
G. Widely split with soft P2
H. Widely split

66. ASD
67. A2 heard before P2; widens on inspiration.
68. Calcific aortic stenosis
69. Left bundle branch block
70. Pulmonary hypertension
71. Pulmonary stenosis
72. Right bundle branch block
73. Systemic hypertension

74. All of the following are causes of late systolic murmurs except:

a) Coarctation of the aorta
b) Acute severe mitral regurgitation
c) Hypertrophic cardiomyopathy
d) Pulmonary arterial stenosis

75. All of the following are causes of early systolic murmurs except:

a) Mitral valve prolapse
b) Papillary muscle rupture
c) Infective endocarditis
d) Rupture of the chordae tendinae

76. Which of the following is LEAST likely to give a thrill on examination?
    a) Acute MR with papillary muscle rupture
    b) VSD
    c) Aortic stenosis
    d) Severe pulmonary insufficiency

77. Which of the following indicates valve mobility in mitral stenosis?
    a) Loud S1
    b) Absence of an opening snap
    c) Loud mid-diastolic murmur
    d) Presence of a mid-systolic click

78. All of the following are considered indicators of severity of mitral stenosis except:
    a) Left atrial enlargement
    b) Abbreviated diastolic murmur
    c) Proximity of opening snap to S2
    d) Presence of a Graham-Steel murmur

79. Which of the following is least likely to be associated with mitral valve prolapse?
    a) Hypertrophic cardiomyopathy
    b) Polyarteritis nodosum
    c) Pseudoxanthoma elasticum
    d) Polycystic ovarian syndrome
    e) Wolff-Parkinson-White syndrome

For the next set of questions match the symptom of aortic stenosis with its average survival/prognosis from time of onset of the symptom. Choose the one BEST answer.

A. 6 months
B. 1 year
C. 2 years
D. 3-5 years

80. Angina

81. Dyspnea

82. Overt cardiac failure

83. Syncope

84. All but which one of the following accurately reflect the current ACC/AHA guidelines for implantation of ICDs (Implantable Cardioverter-Defibrillator)?
   a) Cardiac arrest due to VF or VT not due to a transient or reversible cause
   b) Spontaneous sustained VT
   c) Syncope of undetermined origin with clinically relevant, hemodynamically significant atrial tachycardia or atrial fibrillation induced at EPS when drug therapy is ineffective, not tolerated, or not preferred
   d) Non-sustained VT with CAD, prior MI, LV dysfunction, and inducible VF or sustained VT at EPS that is not suppressible by a class I antiarrhythmic.

85. All of the following are known to increase the risk of sudden death post-MI except:
   a) Low ejection fraction (<30%)
   b) Presence of late potentials on a signal-averaged EKG
   c) Presence of coronary artery disease
   d) Presence of moderate-to-severe dyspnea
   e) Sustained VT or VF from 3 days to 8 weeks following the MI

86. Which of the following is *not* considered an adverse prognostic finding in exercise stress testing?
   a) Prolonged ST segment depression (>3 minutes) after exercise
   b) Peak heart rate < 120 per minute without a pacemaker
   c) Marked ST segment depression (>2mm)
   d) A drop in systolic blood pressure by > 10 mm Hg from baseline

87. Which of the following is not a feature of Cardiac Syndrome X?
   a) Exercise-induced chest pain, so + EST
   b) Atypical features of chest pain (e.g. prolonged episodes, poor response to sublingual nitrates)
   c) Abnormal pain perception in many patients
   d) Poor prognosis regarding survival

88. All of the following are considered features of valvular hemolysis except:
   a) Signs of gross (para)valvular regurgitation
   b) Positive Coombs' test
   c) Normochromic normocytic anemia
   d) Schistocytes on peripheral smear

89. Each of the following is an indication for porcine valve except:
   a) Elderly patient in NSR with normal size left atrium requiring MVR
   b) Elderly patient requiring AVR
   c) Young woman desiring pregnancy
   d) Any patient who can tolerate anticoagulation

90. All but one of the following pairs are considered to have an important drug-drug interaction. Which pair is the exception?
    a) Warfarin and erythromycin
    b) Vasotec and verapamil
    c) Digoxin and quinidine
    d) Verapamil and intravenous beta-blockers

91. All of the following are known arrhythmias in digoxin toxicity except:
    a) Mobitz I
    b) PAT with 2:1 block
    c) Sino-atrial exit block
    d) Mobitz II

92. Which of the following is not a characteristic feature of sick sinus syndrome?
    a) 'Tachy-brady' syndrome (backround sinus tachycardia punctuated by periods of sinus arrest)
    b) Profound sinus arrhythmia with symptoms of tissue hypoperfusion
    c) Periods of sinus arrest (>3s)
    d) Junctional escape rhythms

93. All of the following are true regarding WPW (Wolff-Parkinson-White) syndrome except:
    a) PAT is by far the most common arrhythmia seen in WPW.
    b) Atrial fibrillation is the second most common arrhythmia seen in WPW.
    c) Digitalis and IV verapamil are excellent choices in treating WPW complicated by atrial fibrillation.
    d) WPW is associated with thyrotoxicosis.

94. All of the following are true regarding the use of digoxin in heart failure except:
    a) Patients who should not receive digoxin include those with advanced AV block or those with asymptomatic heart failure.
    b) The benefits of digoxin are greatest in patients with symptomatic CHF, no S3, and a normal heart size.
    c) In general digoxin should be avoided in the acute phase after MI.
    d) Digoxin *may not* be effective in patients who have normal LV systolic function.

95. All of the following are true regarding the latest recommendations for the use of beta-blockers in CHF except:
    a) Nearly all patients with heart failure are considered candidates for β-blockers, as beta-blockers are now considered standard therapy.
    b) Most patients with diabetes can safely use β-blockers.
    c) PVD is a known contraindication to the use of β-blockers.
    d) Initiate β-blocker in CHF only after patient is stable on an ACEI, digoxin, and a diuretic.

For the next set of questions match each cardiomyopathy with the most appropriate management from the options given.

A. Enalapril, hydrochlorothiazide, digoxin, heart transplant
B. Metoprolol or verapamil; dual-chamber pacemaker
C. Diuretics, heart transplant

96. Restrictive cardiomyopathy in a diabetic with amyloidosis
97. Hypertrophic cardiomyopathy
98. Dilated cardiomyopathy in an alcoholic

99. Indications for right heart catheterization include all of the following except:
    a) Uncertainty about the patient's volume status
    b) Comorbid conditions, including ongoing ischemia, sepsis, renal insufficiency, or severe lung disease.
    c) Lack of response to empiric therapy.
    d) Check for patency of the right coronary artery and its tributaries

100. Features distinguishing cardiac tamponade from constrictive pericarditis include all of the following except:
    a) Prominent y-descent
    b) Prominent x-descent
    c) Pericardial knock
    d) Pulsus paradoxus
    e) Kussmaul sign

101. Of all of the following, which is the most important Goldman criteria (preoperative cardiac risk factors for non-cardiac surgery)?
    a) Age > 70
    b) MI within 6 months
    c) S3 gallop
    d) Emergency vascular surgery.

For the next set of questions match the drug with its antiarrhythmic class.

A. Class I
B. Class II
C. Class III
D. Class IV

102. Amiodarone, sotalol
103. Diltiazem, verapamil
104. Metoprolol, propranolol
105. Procainamide

106. All of the following should be routinely checked when screening patients on amiodarone therapy except:
   a) Liver function tests
   b) BUN, creatinine
   c) Pulmonary function tests
   d) TSH and free T4
   e) Slit-lamp examination

107. All of the following are useful features in differentiating HCM from aortic stenosis except:
   a) Double impulse apex beat (HCM)
   b) Late systolic (not ejection) murmur in HCM
   c) Murmur decreases in HCM to valsalva/standing/nitrates
   d) Premature history of sudden death in the family

108. Which of the following is *not* considered in the differential of electromechanical dissociation?
   a) Hypotension
   b) Acidemia, alkalemia
   c) Tamponade
   d) Sino-atrial exit block

For the next set of questions match these commonly used thrombolytic agents with their features.

A. TPA
B. Streptokinase
C. Urokinase

109. APSAK is metabolized to this thrombolytic after injection.

110. Preferentially activates plasminogen, which is adsorbed onto fibrin clots. This serves to direct and localize the lytic process to sites that contain fibrin thrombi. In so doing, it has a high affinity for fibrin and therefore clot specificity.

111. Combines with circulating plasminogen to form a proteolytic complex

112. Commonly causes hypotension

113. A bacterial enzyme

114. A product of renal tubular epithelial cells

115. All of the following are known features of carvedilol (Coreg®) except:
  a) A non-selective β-blocker
  b) An α_1-blocker
  c) Ability to increase the ejection fraction in patients with CHF
  d) Shown to reduce morbidity (though not mortality) in CHF patients.

116. Which of the following is least true regarding verapamil?
  a) Most common side effect is diarrhea.
  b) It should be avoided in patients with sick sinus syndrome as well as those with 2nd or 3rd degree block.
  c) It should be avoided with CHF when the ejection fraction is <40%.
  d) It increases digoxin levels when used simultaneously.

117. Each of the following accurately describes primary hyperaldosteronism except:
  a) Excess aldosterone leads to HTN and ↓ K+ and ↓ renin.
  b) It should be suspected in patients with spontaneous ↓K+ or precipitated by usual dose diuretic therapy.
  c) Diagnosis may be had after a 3-day low salt diet, by measuring Na+, K+, creatinine, and aldosterone in a 24 h urine.
  d) For hyperplastic etiologies (i.e. no mass seen on adrenal CT), treatment is spironolactone.

118. All of the following are true statements about hypertension in pregnancy except:
  a) Preeclampsia includes the triad of hypertension, edema, and proteinuria developing after the 20th week.
  b) A useful differentiator of preeclampsia and chronic hypertension in pregnancy is the increased uric acid often seen in preeclampsia.
  c) Warning signs in ecclampsia include headache, blurry vision, epigastric pain, hyperreflexia, or cerebral symptoms.
  d) Methyldopa is the recommended initial therapy for hypertension in pregnancy. ACE inhibitors may be used instead for patients unable to tolerate methyldopa.

119. Choose the statement that is least true from the following statements regarding the use of nitroprusside in malignant hypertension.
  a) May result in cyanotoxicity if thiocyanate levels are not checked Q72 hours.
  b) Signs and/or symptoms of thiocyanate toxicity include: ataxia; blurred vision; delirium; dizziness; headache; loss of consciousness; nausea and vomiting; shortness of breath; tinnitus.
  c) Na^+Nitrate and hydroxycobalamin (methylene blue) are used to treat toxicity.
  d) Side effects of nitroprusside in general include nausea/vomiting, agitation, flushing, fasciculations and tremor.

For the next set of questions match each condition with the correct renin state.

A. ↑ Renin state
B. ↓ Renin state
C. Either A or B
D. Neither A nor B

120. Bartter's syndrome
121. Beta-blockers, clonidine, methyldopa
122. Cushing's syndrome
123. Diuretics, estrogens, vasodilators
124. End-stage renal disease
125. Essential hypertension
126. Pregnancy
127. Primary hyperaldosteronism
128. Renovascular hypertension

For the next set of questions match each feature with the correct type of hyperlipidemia. Answers may be used once, more than once, or not at all.

A. Type I
B. Type IIA
C. Type IIB
D. Type III
E. Type IV
F. Type V

129. Abnormal Apo E
130. Deficiency of LDL receptors or overproduction of Apo B
131. Deficiency of LPLa (lipoprotein lipase)
132. Eruptive xanthomas, pancreatitis, and CAD
133. Mixed features of Types I + IV
134. Overproduction of Apo B and VLDL
135. Palmar and tuberous xanthomas
136. Reduction in LDL and VLDL receptors
137. Tendon xanthomas

For this next set match each class of lipoprotein with its main role.

A. Chylomicrons
B. VLDL
C. LDL
D. HDL

138. Transport of cholesterol from peripheral cells
139. Transport of cholesterol to peripheral cells
140. Transport of dietary fat
141. Transport of endogenous triglyceride

For the next set of questions, match each secondary cause of hyperlipidemia to A or B.

A. Triglycerides raised
B. Triglycerides *and* cholesterol raised

142. Alcoholism
143. Chronic renal failure
144. Diabetes
145. Estrogen therapy
146. Hypothyroidism
147. Liver disease
148. Nephrotic syndrome
149. Obesity
150. Peritoneal dialysis
151. Renal transplantation

For questions #1-4, match the appropriate recommendation for TB prophylaxis with INH for each situation below. Choose one best answer.

A = INH prophylaxis for induration $\geq$ 5 mm
B = INH prophylaxis for induration $\geq$ 10mm
C = INH prophylaxis for induration $\geq$ 15mm

1. 33yo stonecutter with type II diabetes who was recently diagnosed with silicosis
2. 25 yo prostitute who is found to be HIV-positive
3. A 51 yo Filipino nurse working as a health care administrator in a prison
4. A 44 yo Caucasian mail sorter for the U.S. postal service.

5. All of the following are included in the differential diagnosis of wheezing plus eosinophilia except:
   a) Allergic bronchopulmonary aspergillosis
   b) Löeffler's syndrome
   c) Polyarteritis nodosum
   d) Churg-Strauss syndrome
   e) Strongyloides

6. All of the following statements are true concerning Goodpasture's syndrome except:
   a) Shortness of breath is typically the initial symptom.
   b) Pulmonary involvement usually precedes renal involvement.
   c) Serum ELISA technique can detect anti-basement membrane antibody.
   d) Plasmapheresis is an important adjunct to immunosuppression in reducing this autoantibody.

7. All of the following statements are true concerning bordetella pertussis except:
   a) It is the bacteria responsible for whooping cough.
   b) It should be ruled out in cases of prolonged bronchitis in older children and adults
   c) It may cause a marked lymphocytosis.
   d) Lomefloxacin is the new and currently recommended treatment.
   e) Treatment is aimed at decreasing the spread of the organism by eradicating nasopharyngeal carriage.

8. All of the following statements are true about Legionnaire's disease except:
   a) Clinically patients present with high fever, cough, diarrhea, and bilateral patchy infiltrates.
   b) Labs reveal elevated sodium and LFTs, and a decrease in phosphorous.
   c) Urine antigen-1 is used in Legionnaire's in diagnosis.
   d) Treatment options include erythromycin $\pm$ rifampin; or fluoroquinolone; or azithromycin.

9. All of the following are true statements about pulmonary medicine except:
   a) Hypertrophic pulmonary osteoarthropathy (HOA) can be caused by non-small cell lung ca.
   b) HOA can be seen on Xrays and bone scan
   c) In massive hemoptysis the cause of death is usually exsanguination
   d) In emphysema, there is a decrease in elastic recoil, and an increase in compliance

10. All of the following are true statements about Chlamydia psittacosis except:
   a) The disease involves asymptomatic avian carriers.
   b) Poultry workers are at increased risk.
   c) The disease manifests with fever, chills, headache, *dry* cough, and stiff neck.
   d) It is also commonly referred to as the TWAR agent.

11. Elevated ACE levels may be seen in all of the following conditions except:
   a) Mycoses
   b) Hyperparathyroidism
   c) Primary Biliary Cirrhosis
   d) Reninoma
   e) TB
   f) Asbestosis

12. Which one of the following is *not* considered a relatively common infection in cystic fibrosis?
   a) Klebsiella
   b) Pseudomonas
   c) Aspergillus
   d) Candida albicans

13. Cystic fibrosis is associated with all of the following complications except:
   a) Azospermia
   b) Infertility
   c) Bronchiectasis
   d) Bronchopulmonary fistulas
   e) Nasal polyposis

14. All of the following interstitial lung diseases predominate in the upper lobes except:
   a) Sarcoidosis
   b) Coal worker's pneumonia
   c) Ankylosing spondylitis
   d) Alpha-1-antitrypsin deficiency

15. All of the following interstitial lung diseases predominate in the lower lobes except:
    a) Silicosis
    b) Usual interstitial pneumonia (UIP)
    c) SLE, scleroderma
    d) BOOP

16. Which of the following interstititial lung diseases is not associated with hyperinflated lungs?
    a) Eosinophilic granuloma
    b) LAM (lymphangiomyomatosis)
    c) Idiopathic pulmonary fibrosis
    d) Cystic fibrosis

17. Which of the following statements regarding alveolar proteinosis (AP) is least likely to be true?
    a) It is a diffuse lung disease with deposition of large amounts of phospholipid (PAS+) within alveoli from overproduction by Type II pneumocytes and defective clearance mechanisms.
    b) There is an increased incidence of AP in patients with immunosuppression, hematologic malignancy, and lymphoma.
    c) There is an increased incidence of opportunistic infections, particularly fungal, including nocardia, cryptococcus, and aspergillus.
    d) Presentation is usually acute with dyspnea on exertion secondary to overwhelming of the alveolar sacs.

18. A 67 yo retired naval shipyard worker presents with complaints of increasing dyspnea. He never smoked in his life. His chest X-ray reveals pleural plaques along the diaphragmatic borders bilaterally. Which of the following is least likely to be true regarding his disease?
    a) Among all the fibers, chrysolite is the most common, and crocidolite (the thinnest, longest fibers) is the most carcinogenic.
    b) There is an increased incidence of small cell and large cell carcinoma.
    c) Pleural disease may manifest as "round atelectasis".
    d) Parietal pleural plaques are usually found from the 6th-9th ribs and tend to spare the apices and costophrenic angles.

19. All of the following are true regarding malignant mesothelioma except:
    a) The latent period is usually 30 years after exposure to asbestos. Five percent of asbestosis workers die of mesothelioma.
    b) There is no relationship to cigarette smoking.
    c) Patients with suspected pleural mesothelioma require a fine needle biopsy to obtain cells for definitive diagnosis.
    d) The median survival is 6-12 months.

20. A 19 yo asthmatic teenager is diagnosed with ABPA (allergic bronchopulmonary aspergillosis). Find the statement that is least likely to be true about her disease.
    a) It is a hypersensitivity lung disease caused by aspergillus antigen.
    b) Central segmental bronchi contain mucous plugs full of aspergillus and eosinophils.
    c) Patients require an aggressive approach with agents like amphotericin B.
    d) The upper lobes are preferentially involved.

21. Find the statement that is least true concerning bronchioloalveolar carcinoma.
    a) Bronchioloalveolar carcinoma is a special form of adenocarcinoma arising from peripheral airways.
    b) The prognosis is excellent if resected when < 3 cm.
    c) Patients usually present with a nagging dry cough.
    d) It is associated with pulmonary fibrosis, not unlike its parent adenocarcinoma.

22. All of the following accurately describe features of either bronchiolitis obliterans (BO) or bronchiolitis obliterans with organizing pneumonia (BOOP) except:
    a) It is generally caused by exposure to toxic fumes, infections, drugs, and connective tissue diseases.
    b) Bronchiolitis obliterans is the primary manifestation of chronic rejection in lung transplants. The onset, usually at least 6 months post-transplant, is often subacute with gradual onset of shortness of breath, viral-type symptoms, or malaise.
    c) Destruction of small airways with obliterative scarring is seen on pathology of BO.
    d) Treatment response is minimal and prognosis is poor in BOOP unless the patient receive a lung transplant.

For the next set of questions on bronchogenic carcinoma, match each of the characteristics to the appropriate histology/diagnosis.

A. Adenocarcinoma
B. Squamous cell carcinoma
C. Small cell carcinoma
D. Large cell carcinoma

23. Also known as "scar carcinoma"
24. Bears the highest 5-yr survival of any type
25. Bronchioalveolar carcinoma is considered a subtype
26. Most common type in nonsmokers
27. Most common type to cause SVC syndrome
28. Most common type to cavitate
29. Most commonly associated with hypercalcemia as a non-metastatic manifestation
30. Most rapid growth
31. Poorest survival
32. Most common tracheal neoplasm in the adult
33. Strongest association with smoking

34. Which of the following statements is not true regarding Caplan's syndrome?

a) It describes rheumatoid lung disease when superimposed on pneumoconiosis
b) Nodules usually develop with joint symptoms.
c) Pulmonary nodules appear independently of nodules elsewhere.
d) Patients are typically seropositive for rheumatoid factor.

35. All of the following are true statements about bronchial carcinoid except:

a) While commonly classified as benign, it is in reality a low-grade malignancy.
b) 90% of tumors classified as adenomas are carcinoids.
c) Most carcinoids occur in central bronchi.
d) Prognosis is usually poor with frequent relapses, yielding an overall 5-yr survival of appoximately 24%.

36. Coal workers pneumoconiosis (CWP) bears all of the following features except:

a) It is acquired through chronic exposure to coal dust (coke and anthracite) 1-micron particles.
b) While the simple form of CWP is usually due to exposure to smaller sized particles, it can progress in the absence of further exposure, unlike PMF.
c) CWP is classified as simple and complicated. The complicated form is due to Progressive Massive Fibrosis and is due to exposure to larger particles usually > 1cm in diameter.
d) Radiologically, CWP is usually seen in the periphery and migrates to the hilum.

37. All of the following accurately describe features of rheumatoid pulmonary disease except:

a) Pulmonary manifestations are more common in men.
b) Nodules are the most common pulmonary manifestation.
c) The nodules are identical to the subcutaneous nodules of RA.
d) Patients with pulmonary manifestations usually have other clinical manifestations of RA.

38. Eosinophilic granuloma shows all of the following characteristics except:
a) Granulomatous infiltration of interstitium by histiocytes
b) Diabetes insipidus in 10-25% of patients
c) Most common in black females 55 yo
d) Regression of disease in most

39. A 29 yo hispanic male presents to the ER after an MVA. He sustained severe injuries with multiple compound fractures to his lower extremities. He is stabilized and then undergoes extensive orthopedic repair of his injuries. The operation goes well. However, on the 3rd day post-op, he develops restlessness, delirium, drowsiness, hypoxia, and then suffers a seizure. All of the following are true regarding the most likely etiology of these complications except:

a) His presentation is highly unusual for a fat embolism.
b) About half the patients with fat embolism have retinal and conjunctival punctate hemorrhages or visible fat in retinal vessels.
c) A petechial rash, prominent in the anterior axillary folds and supraclavicular fossae, diffuse interstitial infiltrates on the chest x-ray, fat in the urine, and/or renal failure may also be seen.
d) Severe reduction in arterial oxygen content is common from widespread lung injury (ARDS).

40. All of the following accurately depict characteristics of Goodpasture's syndrome except:

a) The anti-glomerular basement membrane antibodies are a Type III reaction
b) Patients with Goodpasture's syndrome are typically young males (5 to 40 years; male-female ratio of 6:1). In contrast, patients presenting during the second peak in the sixth decade rarely suffer lung hemorrhage and have an almost equal sex distribution. The most common presenting feature is hemoptysis.
c) Most patients have a viral prodrome
d) Most patients present with hypertension.

41. All of the following are true regarding hamartomas except:

a) They are usually asymptomatic and discovered incidentally on routine CXR as a solitary pulmonary nodule.
b) They tend to be well-circumscribed.
c) "Popcorn" calcification is classic, though not common at all.
d) Detection of fat, usually by computerized tomography, is fairly non-specific.

42. All of the following are known features of Hypersensitivity Pneumonitis (extrinsic allergic alveolitis) except:
    a) Pulmonary function studies in all forms of HP typically show a restrictive pattern with loss of lung volumes, impaired diffusion capacity, decreased compliance, and an exercise-induced hypoxemia. A resting hypoxemia may be found.
    b) There are a wide array of agents implicated as causative in HP. Farmer's lung, caused by thermophilic actinomycetes, and found in moldy hay, grain, or silage, is only one of many forms of HP. Other common sources of causative antigens are pet birds as well as heating, cooling, and humidification systems.
    c) Bronchoalveolar lavage in patients with HP consistently demonstrates an increase in macrophages in lavage fluid.
    d) Examination for serum precipitins against suspected antigens is an important part of the diagnostic workup.

43. All of the following are true regarding metastatic disease to the lungs except:
    a) 80% are found in the lung periphery.
    b) Breast, skeletal, and renal primaries account for 80% of mets to the lungs.
    c) The lower lobes are more commonly involved secondary to the distribution of blood flow
    d) Cavitating mets are classically from adenocarcinoma, while >75% of lymphangitic mets are accounted for by squamous.

44. Which of the following is not a correct association with thymoma?
    a) Thymoma (and/or myasthenia gravis) is/are associated with bullous pemphigoid.
    b) 15% of patients with myasthenia gravis have thymoma.
    c) 30% of patients with thymoma have myasthenia gravis.
    d) Thymoma may be present in up to one-third of cases of pure red cell aplasia.

45. Kartagener's (immotile cilia) syndrome and cystic fibrosis share all of the following clinical features except:
    a) Bronchiectasis
    b) Infertility
    c) Pancreatic insufficiency
    d) Sinusitis

46. Patients with obstructive sleep apnea may manifest each of the following symptoms except:
    a) Anemia of chronic disease
    b) Ventricular arrhythmias
    c) Elevated pCO_2
    d) Peripheral edema

47. After a workup including PFTs and bronchoscopy with biopsy, a 49 yo woman is diagnosed with idiopathic pulmonary fibrosis (IPF). All of the following are characteristics of this disease except:

    a) BAL (Bronchoalveolar lavage) can be useful in distinguishing IPF from sarcoidosis. Neutrophils predominate in IPF; whereas lymphocytes predominate in sarcoidosis.
    b) Hypoxemia paradoxically improves with exercise, and PFTs show a restrictive pattern with ↓ DL_{CO} .
    c) Honeycombing on CXR, if seen, is significant, since it signifies advanced disease.
    d) Prognosis is poor without lung transplantation.

48. A 30 yo black female presents with cough, uveitis, hypercalcemia, and erythema nodosum. All of the following are true regarding her most likely disease except:

    a) Only half of these patients have symptoms.
    b) Elevated serum ACE level is diagnostic in the presence of hilar adenopathy.
    c) The presence of non-caseating granulomas is not diagnostic.
    d) Hypergammaglobulinemia, lymphocytopenia, and anergy may be noted on workup.

49. Which of the following stage of sarcoidosis is not correctly defined below?

    a) Stage I: Hilar lymphadenopathy (LN)
    b) Stage II: Hilar LN + pulmonary parenchymal disease
    c) Stage III: Hilar LN + pulmonary parenchymal fibrosis
    d) Stage IV: Pulmonary fibrosis with bullae

50. All of the following are indications for steroids in the management of sarcoidosis except:

    a) Pancreatic calcification
    b) Ocular involvement
    c) Progressive pulmonary disease
    d) Hypercalciuria with renal insufficiency

51. All of the following are examples of eosinophilic pneumonias except:
    a) ABPA
    b) Löeffler's syndrome
    c) Churg-Strauss syndrome
    d) Invasive amebiasis

52. A 45 yo stone cutter, who spent most of his life in the construction business creating tunnels, presents with dyspnea on exertion and progressive pulmonary fibrosis. All of the following are true for his disease except:
    a) There is no increased risk of lung carcinoma.
    b) CXR may show "eggshell" calcifications of the hilar lymph nodes.
    c) If fever is seen, superimposed pulmonary abscess should be suspected.
    d) The disease may be rapidly progressive despite removal from exposure source.

53. Which of the following statements is *least* accurate regarding exercise-induced asthma?
    a) Short-acting β-agonists are first-line therapy.
    b) Cromolyn and nedocromil are effective when taken immediately before the exercise regimen.
    c) Leukotriene inhibitors have been shown to be beneficial in approximately 75% of patients.
    d) Non pharmacological approaches to treatment include a pre-exercise warm-up, exercising in warm, humid air, and exercising in short bursts.

54. Which of the following patterns of calcification of a pulmonary nodule is *not* considered virtually always benign?
    a) Popcorn
    b) Eccentric
    c) Laminated
    d) Central
    e) Diffuse

For the following set of questions, match each pulmonary toxicity to the drug or drugs with which it is associated. Choose the one best answer only from among those listed.

A. Hydralazine
B. Narcotics
C. 'Crack' cocaine
D. Busulfan, bleomycin, BCNU
E. Methotrexate
F. Steroids may predispose
G. Methylsergide
H. Salicylate overdose
I. Prolonged O2 at high FIO_2

55. ARDS
56. Central stimulation of respiratory center leads to respiratory alkalosis
57. Diffuse alveolar hemorrhage, BO$\pm$OP, hypersensitivity pneumonitis
58. Granulomas, endocarditis
59. Hypereosinophilia, hilar lymphadenopathy

60. Nocardia; mycoses
61. Pulmonary fibrosis
62. Retroperitoneal fibrosis
63. SLE-like picture with pleural effusions/pulmonary infiltrates/pleurisy

For the next set of questions, match the macroscopic appearance of each sputum to the most appropriate diagnosis.

A. Amebic abscess
B. Coalworker's pneumoconiosis with progressive, severe fibrosis
C. Alveolar cell carcinoma
D. TB
E. CHF
F. Lung abscess; bronchiectasis
G. Allergic bronchopulmonary aspergillosis
H. Pneumococcal pneumonia

64. Rubbery brown plugs
65. Black
66. Clear, watery, copious
67. Rusty, mucoid
68. Purulent, malodorous
69. Frank blood with simultaneous mucopurulent sputum
70. 'Anchovy sauce'
71. Pink, frothy

72. All of the following are true statements regarding COPD except:
    a) FEV_1 is the most sensitive measure of early airflow obstruction.
    b) To diagnose reversible obstructive lung disease (e.g. asthma), the following parameters should ↑ in response to bronchodilators: FEV_1 or FVC by $\geq$15% or FEF 25-75 by $\geq$ 50%.
    c) A sudden ↓ in the FEV_1 by $\geq$ 20% is an indication for hospitalization.
    d) In patients with COPD, exercise tolerance correlates more with FEV_1, in general, than with their pO_2.

73. Each of the following is considered a major category for the differential diagnosis of an elevated A-a (Alveolar-arterial) gradient except:
    a) V/Q mismatch
    b) Pulmonary vascular disease (e.g. PE)
    c) Shunt
    d) Diffusion defect

74. The differential diagnosis of an increased DL_{CO} include all of the following except:
    a) Mitral stenosis
    b) Polycythemia
    c) Primary pulmonary hypertension
    d) Acute asthma

75. All of the following are in the differential diagnosis of a $\downarrow DL_{CO}$ except:
    a) Goodpasture's syndrome
    b) Idiopathic pulmonary fibrosis
    c) Congestive heart failure
    d) Sarcoidosis

76. Common causes of transudative effusions include all of the following except:
    a) Low albumin states
    b) Empyema
    c) Constrictive pericarditis
    d) Superior vena cava syndrome

77. Other than rheumatoid arthritis, pleural effusions that commonly yield a low pleural fluid glucose include all of the following except:
    a) Empyema
    b) Malignancy
    c) Esophageal rupture
    d) Tuberculosis

78. Which of the following is *not* included among the known age-related changes in pulmonary function?
    a) $\downarrow$ FEV
    b) $\uparrow$ pCO_2
    c) $\uparrow$ FRC (forced residual capacity)
    d) $\downarrow$ pO_2
    e) $\downarrow$ VC (vital capacity)

79. All of the following are true regarding α-1 antitrypsin deficiency except:
    a) There is experimental evidence that the structural integrity of lung elastin depends on this antienzyme, which protects the lung from proteases released from leukocytes.
    b) Most members of the normal population have two M genes, designated as protease inhibitor type MM, and have serum α1AT levels in excess of 2.5 g/L.
    c) The emphysema in α1AT deficiency is a panacinar process that predominates in the upper lung fields.
    d) Liver transplantation restores normal levels of this enzyme and so appears to play a critical role in this disease.

80. Which of the following is an accurate statement regarding the value of the D-dimer assay in the workup of pulmonary embolus?
    a) For patients with a high clinical suspicion of disease, an elevated D-dimer result can spare the patient the unnecessary risk of a pulmonary angiogram.
    b) For patients with a low pretest probability of disease, an elevated D-dimer provides a strong argument for anticoagulating based on an indeterminate V/Q scan.
    c) For patients with a high pretest probability of disease, an elevated D-dimer has a positive predictive value of 98%.
    d) For patients with a low pretest probability of disease, a normal D-dimer assay has a negative predictive value of 99%.

81. All of the following are potential pulmonary complications of rheumatoid arthritis except:
    a) Caplan's syndrome
    b) Spontaneous pulmonary hemorrhage
    c) Obliterative bronchiolitis
    d) Bronchopulmonary fistula
    e) Pulmonary hypertension

82. All of the following slow the rate of elimination of theophylline except:
    a) CHF
    b) Smoking
    c) Obesity
    d) Oral contraceptives
    e) Erythromycin

83. Which of the following is not considered a characteristic of chronic eosinophilic pneumonia?
    a) Central pulmonary infiltrates
    b) Asthma and BOOP are known associations.
    c) Eosinophilia is seen in the tissue *and* blood.
    d) Responds favorably to steroids.

84. A 27 yo male presents in acute respiratory failure following a serious motor vehicle accident. He is placed on assist control mechanical ventilation with an FIO_2 of 80%, a backup rate of 20, a Tidal Volume of 800cc, and no PEEP. The first gas on these settings comes back and shows good ventilation, but the pO_2 is 310 and the saturation is 100%. What is the appropriate adjustment that needs to be made in his ventilator settings?
    a) Reduce the FIO_2 to 27%
    b) Reduce the FIO_2 to 44%
    c) Reduce the FIO_2 to 50%
    d) Reduce the FIO_2 to 65%

85. Each of the following is a list of potential benefits that PEEP can have on cardiopulmonary function except:
    a) It prevents alveolar collapse.
    b) It plays an important role in recruiting collapsed alveolar units.
    c) It allows one to limit oxygen toxicity from prolonged FIO_2 above 60%.
    d) It improves cardiac output by 2-3%.

86. All of the following are considered weaning criteria in mechanical ventilation except:
    a) FIO_2 <40%
    b) NIF (negative inspiratory force) $\geq$ 25
    c) PEEP <5
    d) PaO_2 >60

For the next set of questions, match each of the following common ventilator problems to the usual/common source of problem. Each answer may be used once only. Choose the one best answer.

A. High peak pressure
B. Low pressure (peak) alarm
C. High peak and plateau pressures
D. Low compliance

87. ARDS
88. Cuff leak/cuff rupture
89. Mucus plugging
90. Pneumothorax; congestive heart failure

91. All of the following are frequently associated with pneumonia and hepatitis except:
    a) Mycoplasma pneumoniae
    b) Chlamydia psittaci
    c) Coxiella burnetti
    d) Klebsiella pneumoniae
    e) Toxoplasmosis

ENDOCRINOLOGY QUESTIONS

1. All of the following are true statements concerning TFM (testicular feminization) except:
   a) These are genetic females affected with ambiguous genitalia.
   b) TFM is also known as "Male pseudohermaphroditism".
   c) Patients with TFM lack the enzyme 5 α-reductase to convert testosterone to DHT, the active form in the tissues.
   d) At adolescence normal breast and female 2° sex characteristics are seen; however pubic hair and menarche are lacking.

2. All of the following are true statements concerning amenorrhea except:
   a) Ovarian disorders are common causes and PCO (polycystic ovarian syndrome) is the most common among these.
   b) PCO is characterized by obesity, hirsutism, amenorrhea, and an FSH/LH ratio >2:1.
   c) Post-pill amenorrhea accounts for 30% of secondary amenorrhea cases.
   d) Drugs, such as phenothiazenes and metoclopramide, may cause amenorrhea by inducing a hyperprolactinemia.

3. In the evaluation of hirsutism, all of the following are true except:
   a) In CAH (congenital adrenal hyperplasia), the LH/FSH ratio is usually > 3:1.
   b) Efforts should be made to locate the source of the androgens. The main sources of androgens are DHEAS, which comes from the adrenals, and testosterone, which comes from the ovaries and adrenals.
   c) Levels of testosterone >200 indicate an ovarian or adrenal neoplasm.
   d) Levels of DHEAS > 7ng/dl usually point toward an adrenal tumor or CAH.

4. All of the following are true statements about congenital adrenal hyperplasia except:
   a) Patients with 17α hydroxylase deficiency are frequently hypertensive.
   b) Patients with 21 hydroxylase deficiency are frequently virilized.
   c) 17α hydroxylase deficiency is the most common form of CAH.
   d) 17 α hydroxyprogesterone is not the only source of androstenedione, as it may also come from DHEA.

5. In the evaluation of amenorrhea, all of the following are true regarding the gonadotropins:
   a) ↑LH and ↑FSH are seen in pregnancy.
   b) ↑FSH is seen in ovarian failure.
   c) ↑LH and ↓FSH are seen in Polycystic Ovarian Syndrome.
   d) ↓LH and ↓FSH are seen in hypopituitarism.

6. All of the following are clinical features associated with acromegaly except:
   a) Carbohydrate intolerance
   b) ↓ cold tolerance
   c) Hyperprolactinemia
   d) Cardiomyopathy
   e) Acanthosis nigricans

Questions # 7-13 are matching-type questions on Diabetes Insipidus. Choose one best answer.

A. Central DI
B. Nephrogenic DI
C. Primary Polydipsia
D. A and B
E. B and C

7. Characterized by decreased production of ADH (antidiuretic hormone)

8. Characterized by decreased responsiveness to ADH

9. Lack of response to the addition of exogenous ADH

10. Lithium can cause DI

11. Positive response to the water deprivation test

12. Treatment includes thiazides

13. Treatment is intranasal dDAVP (desmopressin)

Questions # 14-18 are matching-type questions concerning thyroiditis. Choose one best answer.

A. Microbial inflammatory thyroiditis
B. Subacute granulomatous thyroiditis
C. Graves' disease
D. Subacute lymphocytic thyroiditis
E. Chronic lymphocytic thyroiditis

14. A patient taking levothyroxine for what he was told was 'Hashimoto's thyroiditis'.

15. Patient presents with neck pain and the RAIU (radioactive iodine uptake) is ↑

16. Patient presents with neck pain and the RAIU (radioactive iodine uptake) is ↓

17. Patient presents with thyrotoxicosis and an ↓ RAIU.

18. Patient presents with thyrotoxicosis and an ↑ RAIU.

Questions # 19-25 are matching-type questions related to subacute and silent thyroiditis. Match the clinical findings to the appropriate diagnosis/diagnoses.

A. Subacute thyroiditis
B. Silent thyroiditis
C. Both A and B
D. Neither A nor B

19. A relatively common form of thyroiditis
20. Painful, tender goiter
21. Disease is self-limiting.
22. Causative agent is felt to be viral.
23. ESR is normal.
24. Often seen postpartum
25. Transient period of thyrotoxicosis may be followed by a short period of hypothyroidism.

For the next set of questions match each ocular finding to its appropriate classification.

A. Infiltrative finding (Graves' disease only)
B. Noninfiltrative finding (any thyrotoxicosis)

26. Extraocular muscle dysfunction
27. Lid lag
28. Lid retraction
29. Optic neuritis
30. Proptosis

31. Which of the following is NOT considered a characteristic laboratory finding in factitious thyrotoxicosis?
    a) High T_4 or T_3
    b) Low serum thyroglobulin
    c) Low TSH
    d) High I^{131} uptake

32. All of the following are potential side effects of propylthiouracil (PTU) except:
    a) Agranulocytosis
    b) Aplastic anemia
    c) Azotemia
    d) Vasculitis

33. Which of the following is NOT a feature of thyroid nodules?
    a) Approximately 90% are benign.
    b) Approximately 10% are 'cold' nodules.
    c) Approximately 90% are solid.
    d) 20% of cold nodules are malignant.

For the next set of questions match each characteristic feature with the correct type of thyroid carcinoma. Choose one best answer.

A. Papillary carcinoma
B. Follicular carcinoma
C. Anaplastic carcinoma
D. Medullary carcinoma

34. Best prognosis
35. Calcitonin is used as a tumor marker
36. May be part of MEN IIA or IIB
37. Most aggressive
38. Spreads via lymph nodes and can present with a thyroid mass and cervical lymphadenopathy
39. Carries the worst prognosis
40. Most common
41. The Hürthle cell tumor is a subtype of this tumor.
42. Classically undergoes early hematogenous spread, and the patient may present with distant metastases.

43. All of the following are correct statements regarding euthyroid sick syndrome except:
    a) Labs generally show a $\downarrow T_3$, $\downarrow T_4$, and $\uparrow$sTSH
    b) Aka "adaptive hypothyroidism"
    c) Commonly seen in sick/hospitalized patients
    d) The condition is primarily a laboratory phenomenon, is only a reflection of the patient's generally ill condition, and warrants no additional treatment.

44. Among the following statements regarding thyrotoxic crisis (TC), find the statement that is least likely to be true.
    a) TC is generally seen in untreated or inadequately treated hyperthyroid patients undergoing surgical treatment or who have another acute illness.
    b) The early clinical presentation includes irritability/restlessness, hyperthermia, tachycardia, hypertension, and vomiting/diarrhea.
    c) PTU (propylthiouracil), sodium iodide, and propranolol are used to control the crisis.
    d) PTU blocks the synthesis of thyroxine, and sodium iodide blocks the release of thyroxine from the thyroid.

45. From the following characteristics concerning myxedema coma, find the feature that is least true.

a) It occurs with severe hypothyroidism.
b) Hyponatremia and hypoglycemia are seen.
c) Aggressive management with IV thyroxine and high dose steroids is warranted.
d) A waxy, pretibial edema is one of the classic signs that may be seen on examination.

46. All of the following are skeletal lesions that can be found in primary hyperparathyroidism except:

a) Subperiosteal bone resorption e.g. at the distal phalanges;
b) Osteomalacia
c) Ostitis fibrosis cystica
d) Salt and pepper lesions seen on skull plain film

47. From the following statements regarding FHH (Familial Hypocalciuric Hypercalcemia), find the incorrect statement.

a) Autosomal dominant hypercalcemia is frequently seen in a relatively young patient.
b) PTH is normal to slightly increased, and therefore, cannot be used to differentiate it from primary hyperparathyroidism, so check the urine calcium.
c) Urine calcium is usually elevated in FHH, making this a great way to differentiate FHH and primary hyperparathyroidism.
d) The diagnosis of FHH is important in the differential of hyperparathyroidism since FHH precludes parathyroidectomy.

48. Each of the statements below is correct regarding calcium metabolism except:

a) Thiazides cause a mild hypercalciuria and, if left unchecked, may lead to symptomatic hypocalcemia.
b) Lithium causes an ↑ serum Ca in 10% of patients by increasing the setpoint of PTH secretion.
c) FHH, thiazides, and lithium are common causes of "normal" or "minimally-elevated" PTH.
d) Hypercalcemia in Addison's, vit D intoxication, and sarcoidosis is steroid-responsive.

Hypercalcemia of malignancy works through several different mechanisms, depending on the type of tumor. For the next set of questions, match the mechanism of hypercalcemia with the types of tumors listed. Choose one best answer.

A. Multiple myeloma
B. Lymphoma
C. Squamous cell carcinoma of the lung/head/neck as well as carcinoma of the breast/GU tract

49. Presence of PTH-rP (PTH-related Protein)
50. OAF (Osteoclast Activating Factor)
51. Ectopic production of 1,25 Vit D

52. All of the following are true regarding hypoparathyroidism except:
    a) Pseudohypoparathyroidism is secondary to end-organ resistance to PTH. Urinary cAMP levels are depressed and PTH is elevated.
    b) The clinical phenotype includes short stature/short neck/short metacarpals; rounded face/obesity/mild mental retardation.
    c) Subcutaneous calcification is another clinical sign that may be seen in pseudohypoparathyroidism.
    d) *Pseudopseudo*hypoparathyroidism is clinically very similar to pseudohypoparathyroidism, but the biochemical markers seen are completely different.

For the next set of questions match each disorder with the appropriate choice of MEN syndrome(s) to which it is commonly attributed from the answers below.

A. MEN I (Wermer syndrome)
B. MEN IIA (Sipple syndrome)
C. MEN IIB
D. Both A & B
E. Both B & C
F. None of the above

53. Pituitary tumors
54. Parathyroid tumors
55. Pancreatic carcinoma
56. Pheochromocytoma
57. Medullary thyroid carcinoma
58. Marfanoid features

For the following set match each disease with the correct Polyglandular Autoimmune (PGA) syndrome(s).

A. PGA I
B. PGA II
C. Both
D. Neither

59. Adrenal insufficiency
60. Alopecia
61. Chronic active hepatitis
62. Graves' disease
63. Hypogonadism
64. Hypoparathyroidism
65. Hypothyroidism
66. Malabsorption
67. Mucocutaneous candidiasis
68. Myasthenia gravis
69. Pernicious anemia
70. Type 1 diabetes
71. Vitiligo

72. What is the currently accepted threshold for a fasting glucose-based diagnosis of diabetes?

    a) 114
    b) 126
    c) 140
    d) 175
    e) 200

73. Respectively, what are the currently accepted glucose levels that are considered "normal" during fasting state and 2 hours into an oral glucose tolerance test?

    a) <114 and < 140
    b) <126 and < 200
    c) <140 and < 175
    d) <110 and < 140

74. Find the statement least likely to be correct from among the following statements regarding the Somogyi effect and the Dawn phenomenon.

    a) The Somogyi effect describes rebound hyperglycemia 2° to counter-regulatory hormones (such as GH) that follows a hypoglycemic episode.
    b) The Dawn phenomenon refers to early AM hyperglycemia 2° to insulin resistance.
    c) Usually, the dawn phenomenon can be differentiated from post-hypoglycemic hyperglycemia by measuring the blood glucose at 3 A.M.
    d) The distinction is considered academic since both involve elevated morning glucose that may be corrected by increasing the evening insulin.

For the following set of questions match the primary action to the appropriate oral hypoglycemic medication.

A. Rosiglitazone, pioglitazone
B. Repaglinide
C. Metformin
D. Miglitol

75. Stimulate pancreatic beta cells to ↑ insulin output
76. Inhibit intestinal enzymes that break down carbohydrates, delaying carbohydrate absorption
77. Bind to peroxisome-proliferator-activated receptor-gamma (PPAR-gamma) in muscle, fat, and liver to ↓ insulin resistance
78. ↓ hepatic glucose production ; ↑ glucose uptake in muscle tissue

79. Complications of proliferative retinopathy include all of the following except:
    a) Vitreous hemorrhage
    b) Neovascularization
    c) Microaneurysms
    d) Retinal detachment

80. Which of the following statements is *not* true about diabetic amyotrophy?
    a) Diabetic amyotrophy is a chronic condition that progresses, though very slowly, over years.
    b) It is likely a form of neuropathy, affecting the proximal major nerve trunks and lumbosacral plexus, although atrophy and weakness of the large muscles in the upper leg and pelvic girdle resemble primary muscle disease.
    c) Anorexia and depression may accompany amyotrophy. Because of the weight loss, such patients are often thought to have a paraneoplastic neuropathy.
    d) More appropriate terms for this disorder include *diabetic proximal neuropathy* and *lumbosacral plexopathy*.

81. All of the following are accurate statements that should be carefully considered when managing a patient with diabetic ketoacidosis except:
   a) As the metabolic acidosis and hyperglycemia correct, serum K+ decreases, so one must remember to add KCl to the IV fluids.
   b) DKA patients are deficient in total body K+ regardless of their plasma K+ concentration.
   c) Remember to switch from IV insulin to SQ when serum glucose decreases to 200-250.
   d) The best way to monitor a patient with DKA for improvement is with urine ketones, and not serial anion gaps.

For the following set of questions match the ACTH level and response to high dose dexamethasone with the correct Cushing's diagnosis.

A. Cushing's disease
B. Cushing's syndrome
C. Ectopic/paraneoplastic Cushing's

82. ↓ACTH and non-suppressible to high dose dexamethasone
83. ↑ACTH and non-suppressible to high dose dexamethasone
84. ↑ACTH and suppressible to high dose dexamethasone

85. Each of the following is a well-known cause of a false-positive dexamethasone suppression test except:
   a) Estrogen, oral contraceptives, or pregnancy
   b) Simple obesity
   c) Depression
   d) Diabetes insipidus
   e) Alcoholism
   f) Hospitalized patients

86. A 33 yo black female is found to have hypercalcemia on routine laboratory testing. Her albumin is 4.5, and an intact PTH is < 81. Thereafter a 25, OH vit D level is found to be 35 (normal). All of the following remain in the differential based on this information alone except:
   a) Hyperthyroidism
   b) Adrenal insufficiency
   c) Milk-alkali syndrome
   d) Sarcoidosis
   e) Thiazides

For the next set of question, match each set of laboratory parameters with the correct cause of hypoglycemia.

A. Sulfonylurea abuse
B. Surreptitious insulin
C. Insulinoma

Q#	Glucose	Insulin	C-peptide	Proinsulin
87.	↓	↑	↑	↔
88.	↓	↑↑	↓	↓
89.	↓	↑	↑	↑

90. An 18 yo female is suspected of having congenital adrenal hyperplasia. For confirmation, levels of 17αhydroxylase, 21-hydroxylase, and 11β-hydroxylase are sent off. When they return only the 17αhydroxylase is deficient. Which of the following physical findings might you expect to find in this individual?
a) Hypertension
b) Edema
c) Hirsutism
d) Hyperkalemia

For the next set of questions match each malignancy to the ectopic hormone with which it may be associated in paraneoplastic phenomena.

A. PTH
B. ACTH
C. Renin

91. Adenocarcinoma of the kidney
92. Breast carcinoma
93. Bronchial carcinoid
94. Lung carcinoma
95. Oat cell carcinoma
96. Squamous cell tumors

NEPHROLOGY QUESTIONS

For the following set of questions, match each feature with the correct type(s) of RTA (renal tubular acidosis) associated with it.

A. Type I
B. Type II
C. Type IV
D. A&B
E. A&C
F. None of the above

1. Amphotericin B
2. Hypokalemia
3. Distal RTA
4. Aminoglycosides
5. Proximal RTA
6. Diabetes
7. Benign prostatic hypertrophy
8. NSAIDs
9. Hyporeninemic hyperaldosteronism

10. All of the following statements are true about metabolic alkalosis except:
    a) A urine chloride should always be ordered in cases of metabolic alkalosis of unclear origin.
    b) A urine chloride < 10 points to surreptitious vomiting.
    c) A urine chloride > 10 points to Bartter's syndrome and diuretics.
    d) Laxative abuse is a form of metabolic alkalosis where urine chloride < 10.

11. All of the following parameters are typical of Bartter's syndrome except:
    a) Blood pressure is normal to high/normal.
    b) Renin is elevated
    c) Aldosterone levels are elevated.
    d) K+ is $\downarrow$
    e) ABG reveals a chloride-resistant metabolic alkalosis.

12. Autosomal Dominant Polycystic Kidney Disease is frequently associated with all of the following except:
    a) Mitral valve prolapse
    b) Hepatic cysts
    c) Myocardial infarction
    d) Elevated hematocrit
    e) Cerebral aneurysms

13. Of all the types of renal calculi, calcium oxalate stones are the most common. They result from all of the following aberrations in the urine except:
    a) Hypercalcemia
    b) Hyperoxaluria
    c) Hypercitraturia
    d) Hyperuricemia

14. A workup for causes of nephrolithiasis is indicated for all of the following except:
    a) A patient with a history of recurrent stones
    b) A patient who reports a positive family history of renal stones
    c) A 24 yo patient who presents with his first stone, only mildly symptomatic
    d) A 32 yo patient who presents with excruciating left flank pain, and gross hematuria, and is subsequently diagnosed with nephrolithiasis.

For the following set of questions, match the disease with the correct histological pattern(s) of glomerular disease. Some diseases have more than one answer.

A. Diffuse proliferative GN
B. Crescentic GN
C. Focal proliferative GN
D. Mesangial proliferative GN
E. Membranoproliferative GN
F. Minimal change GN
G. Focal segmental GN
H. Nodular sclerosis
I. Membranous GN
J. Deposition disease
K. Thrombotic microangiopathy

15. Amyloid
16. Cryoglobulinemia
17. Diabetic nephropathy
18. Drug-induced interstitial nephritis
19. Goodpasture's syndrome
20. Henoch-Schönlein purpura/ IgA nephropathy
21. Hepatitis B & C
22. Heroine use
23. HIV
24. Hodgkin's lymphoma
25. Immune complex GN
26. Malignant hypertension
27. Pauci-immune GN
28. Penicillamine, captopril
29. Post-transplant (renal, bone marrow)
30. SBE
31. Solid organ neoplasms

For the next set of questions, match each glomerular disease with the appropriate target of injury.

A. Endothelial cell
B. Mesangial cell
C. Basement membrane
D. Visceral epithelial cell
E. Parietal epithelial cell

33. Acute renal failure
34. Crescentic GN
35. Membranous nephropathy
36. Mesangioproliferative GN/glomerulosclerosis
37. Minimal change disease and focal segmental glomerular sclerosis
38. Thrombotic microangiopathies

39. All of the following diseases are associated with IgA nephropathy except:
    a) Celiac disease
    b) Obstructive bronchiolitis
    c) Graves' disease
    d) Mycosis fungoides
    e) Ankylosing spondylitis

For the following set of questions match each disorder with the appropriate immunofluorescence microscopy findings.

A. Linear Ig and C3
B. Sparse or absent Ig/C3
C. Granular Ig and C3 (low C3)
D. Granular Ig and C3 (normal C3)

40. Atheroemboli
41. Bacterial endocarditis
42. Cryoglobulinemia
43. Goodpasture's syndrome
44. HUS/TTP
45. IgA nephropathy/Henoch-Schönlein purpura
46. Interstitial nephritis
47. Lupus nephritis
48. Malignant HTN
49. Microscopic polyarteritis nodosa
50. Membranoproliferative GN
51. Postinfectious GN
52. Scleroderma crisis
53. Wegener's granulomatosis

For this next set match each drug with the glomerular lesion it can induce.

A. Minimal change disease
B. Membranous nephropathy
C. Focal segmental glomerulosclerosis
D. Pauci-immune necrotizing GN
E. Proliferative GN with vasculitis
F. Rapidly progressive GN

54. Allopurinol
55. Alpha-interferon
56. Amoxicillin
57. Ampicillin
58. Captopril
59. Ciprofloxacin
60. Heroin
61. NSAIDs
62. Penicillamine
63. Penicillin
64. Rifampin
65. Sulfonamides
66. Thiazides
67. Warfarin

For the next set match each characteristic to the MOST appropriate disease involving renal tubular defects. Choose the one best answer.

A. Autosomal dominant polycystic kidney disease
B. Autosomal recessive polycystic kidney disease
C. Tuberous sclerosis
D. Medullary sponge kidney
E. Medullary cystic disease
F. Liddle's syndrome
G. Bartter's syndrome
H. RTA, Type I
I. RTA, Type II
J. RTA, Type IV

68. Chronic renal insufficiency; reduced proton and potassium secretion
69. Congenital hepatic fibrosis
70. Dilated collecting ducts; nephrocalcinosis; hematuria

71. Hepatic cysts; intracranial aneurysms; colonic diverticuli
72. Hyperplasia of the juxtaglomerular apparatus; hypokalemia, alkalosis, and high aldosterone levels
73. Hypokalemia, alkalosis, low aldosterone levels, and hypertension
74. Medullary cysts; small kidneys
75. Nephrocalcinosis; impaired proton secretion in the distal tubule; non-anion-gap metabolic acidosis
76. Reduced bicarbonate reabsorption, non-anion-gap metabolic acidosis; Fanconi syndrome
77. Renal cysts and angiomyolipomas

For this next set of questions match each feature to the correct non-anion gap acidosis/acidoses from the choices given. Choose ALL answers that apply.

A. Type I RTA
B. Type II RTA
C. Type IV RTA
D. GI bicarbonate loss

78. Daily acid excretion is low
79. Daily bicarbonate needs are generally >4 mmol/kg
80. Fanconi syndrome
81. Minimum urine pH <5.5
82. Nephrolithiasis/nephrocalcinosis
83. Positive urine anion gap
84. Serum K+ is low

85. Both poststreptococcal GN (PSGN) and IgA nephropathy frequently follow upper respiratory infection. How can one clinically differentiate between the two?

    a) PSGN is typically much more severe.
    b) PSGN typically precedes IgA nephropathy by 1-2 weeks.
    c) PSGN occurs 7-21 days after the URI, versus 3 days in IgA nephropathy.
    d) Urine potassium is usually elevated in IgA nephropathy, and not in PSGN.

86. All of the following are associated with hypomagnesemia except:

    a) Bartter's syndrome
    b) Cyclosporine
    c) Hyperparathyroidism
    d) Cisplatinum

For the following group of questions, match the findings on sediment analysis with the type of acute renal failure in which it is most commonly found. Choose one BEST answer.

A. Prerenal azotemia
B. Tubular injury
C. Interstitial nephritis
D. Glomerulonephritis

87. Hyaline casts
88. Pigmented granular casts
89. RBC, RBC casts
90. WBC, WBC casts, eosinophils, eosinophil casts

91. All of the following types of renal stones are known to form in acid urine except:
    a) Struvite stones
    b) Uric acid stones
    c) Calcium oxalate stones
    d) Cystine stones

For the next set of questions, choose the renal disorder with which the given drug(s) is (are) associated.

A. Prerenal azotemia
B. ATN (acute tubular necrosis)
C. Intratubular obstruction
D. Rhabdomyolysis
E. Membranous GN
F. FSGN (focal segmental GN)
G. Urolithiasis
H. Retroperitoneal fibrosis
I. HUS (Hemolytic Uremic Syndrome)
J. Acute interstitial nephritis
K. Chronic renal failure
L. Nephrogenic DI
M. Hyperkalemia
N. Hyponatremia
O. Hypomagnesemia
P. Hypocalcemia
Q. Hypokalemia

92. β-lactam antibiotics; sulfonamides; diuretics
93. ACE inhibitors
94. Acyclovir, methotrexate
95. Allopurinol
96. Aminoglycosides

97. Amphotericin
98. Aspirin; acetaminophen
99. Cysplatin
100. Heroin
101. Lithium
102. Lovastatin; gemfibrozil
103. Methylsergide
104. Mitomycin C
105. Penicillamine
106. Radiocontrast
107. Thiazides

1. Anion gap metabolic acidoses are caused by all of the following except:
   a) Propylene glycol
   b) Isopropyl alcohol
   c) Iron
   d) Isoniazid
   e) Strychnine

2. A 33 yo intravenous drug abuser presents with miosis, respiratory depression, and drowsiness. The ER physician diagnoses him with opiate overdose. By the time the patient hits the medical ward, the patient is still quite lethargic. The opiate level is back and is markedly positive as suspected. Your next step in management is...
   a) Counsel the patient to voluntarily enter a drug rehabilitation center.
   b) Give the patient a bolus dose of naloxone. Once he wakes up and is fully oriented and feeling better, he can be discharged with follow-up with his primary care physician.
   c) Give the patient a test dose IV push of naloxone. Once he wakes up and is fully oriented and feeling better, place him on an IV naloxone drip, and continue to monitor him for the next 24 hours.
   d) Give the patient a bolus dose of naloxone. Once he wakes up and is fully oriented and feeling better, he can be sent home on PO methadone to follow-up on his own volition at the drug rehabilitation center.

3. All of the following statements are true in toxicology except:
   a) Methanol and ethylene glycol cause both an elevated anion gap and an elevated osmolar gap.
   b) In addition to activated charcoal, salicylate poisonings are best handled thru use of fluids, monitoring K+ levels, and alkalinizing the urine.
   c) Charcoal is generally effective in absorbing alcohols and lithium.
   d) Charcoal should not be given in cases of suspected caustic ingestions.

For question # 4-12 match each antidote with the appropriate drug/toxin.

A. Anticholinergics
B. Benzodiazepines
C. Beta-blockers
D. Cyanide
E. Ethylene glycol
F. Narcotics
G. Nitrites
H. Organophosphates
I. Tricyclic antidepressants

4. Amyl nitrite
5. Atropine, pralidoxamine
6. Ethanol

7. Flumazenil
8. Glucagon
9. Methylene blue
10. Naloxone
11. Physostigmine
12. Sodium bicarbonate

13. In managing digoxin overdose, all of the following are true except:
    a) Atropine is often effective for bradycardias.
    b) Lidocaine and dilantin are contraindicated as they may induce ventricular irritability.
    c) Digoxin-specific Fab fragments (Digibind®) are reserved only for severe intoxication.
    d) Digoxin levels are unreliable following treatment with Digibind.

14. Each of the following statements is true regarding tricyclic antidepressant overdose except:
    a) It accounts for approximately 3% of all deaths due to poisoning.
    b) Seizures are a common complication.
    c) Activated charcoal is an important treatment.
    d) For hypotension isuproterenol, dobutamine, or low-dose dopamine may be used.

BLOOD GAS ANALYSIS QUESTIONS

1. If PaO_2 *does not* correct with an increase in the FIO_2 %, all of the following are potential diagnoses *except*:
   a) Atelectasis
   b) Aspiration
   c) Pulmonary hemorrhage
   d) Pulmonary embolus

2. A patient presents with the following blood gas: pH 7.55, pCO_2 54, pO_2 88, HCO_3^- 34, and oxygen sat of 94%. What is the next step in the analysis of this patient's potential diagnoses?
   a) Calculate the A-a gradient
   b) Check the chemistries for an osmolar gap
   c) Check the urine chloride
   d) Check the urine potassium

3. A urine chloride of less than 10 is MOST consistent with which of the following diagnoses?
   a) Diarrhea
   b) Bartter's syndrome
   c) Hyperaldosteronism
   d) Cushing's syndrome

4. All of the following are potential diagnoses in a patient with a low PaO_2 that improves with an increase in the FIO_2% except:
   a) Asthma
   b) Pneumonia
   c) Interstitial lung disease
   d) Pulmonary embolus

5. What is the meaning of the "delta-delta" equation in the study of acid-base disorders?
   a) It is the change in anion gap divided by the change in the bicarbonate.
   b) It is the deviation of the measured osmolar gap from normal minus the deviation of the anion gap from normal.
   c) It is a formulaic expression of the Winter's formulas relating to chronic respiratory processes.
   d) It is an direct measure of the difference in expected bicarbonate from the calculated bicarbonate using the Winter's formulas.

6. What is the important cut-off level, clinically, for the delta-delta?
   a) ½
   b) 1
   c) 2
   d) 3

7. What is the meaning of a delta delta >1 ?
   a) There is a concealed metabolic alkalosis.
   b) There is a concealed non-anion gap metabolic acidosis.
   c) There is a concealed osmolar gap.
   d) The patient is not compensating sufficiently.

8. If a patient's anion gap is 20 and her measured HCO_3- is 19, what is going on?
   a) There is a concealed metabolic alkalosis.
   b) There is a concealed non-anion gap metabolic acidosis.
   c) There is a concealed osmolar gap.
   d) The patient is not compensating sufficiently.

9. What is the number one cause of hypoxemia?
   a) Abnormal lungs
   b) Pneumonia
   c) Atelectasis
   d) Hypoventilation

For the following set of questions match each situation with the most likely diagnosis.

A. Leukocyte larceny
B. Methemoglobinemia
C. Cyanide poisoning or carboxyhemoglobinemia

10. Percent saturation is unusually high for the level of PaO_2
11. A low PaO_2, a low % saturation on the blood gas, and a normal pulse oximetry in a non-cyanotic patient
12. Low saturation yet normal PaO_2 in a cyanotic patient

For the next set of questions match the acid-base disorder(s) with the correct way to calculate appropriate compensation.

A. Metabolic acidosis
B. Metabolic alkalosis
C. Respiratory acidosis/ alkalosis

13. Expected HCO_3- is calculated using formulas based on measured pCO_2.
14. Expected pCO_2=1.5(HCO_3-) + 8 ± 2
15. Rule of thumb whereby the last 2 digits equals the last 2 digits of the pH.

For the next set of questions match each set of acid-base parameters with the correct clinical scenario.

A. Arterial hypoxemia from a V/Q mismatch without a right-to-left shunt
B. CarboxyHgb, cyanide poisoning, malignant hyperthermia, status epilepticus.
C. Erythrocytosis 2° to obstructive sleep apnea (nocturnal hypoxemia)
D. Intracardiac or intrapulmonary right-to-left shunt
E. Leukocyte larceny 2° leukemia
F. Methemoglobinemia with congenital right-shifted hemoglobin
G. Normal lungs with a respiratory acidosis
H. Normal lungs with a respiratory alkalosis
I. Respiratory acidosis in a patient with abnormal lungs
J. Respiratory alkalosis in a patient with abnormal lungs
K. Venous blood sample

16. ↓ PaO_2, $PaCO_2$ 47, normal pulse ox
17. ↑ PaO_2, ↓ $PaCO_2$, normal A-a gradient
18. ↓ PaO_2, ↑ $PaCO_2$, normal A-a gradient
19. Normal or ↓ PaO_2, ↓ $PaCO_2$, ↑ A-a gradient
20. Normal paO_2 and sat but increased Hgb
21. ↓ PaO_2 and sat, $PaCO_2$ normal/↓, ↑gradient, PaO_2 corrects with ↑ FIO_2%
22. ↓ PaO_2 and sat, $PaCO_2$ normal/↓, ↑gradient, PaO_2 does not correct with ↑ FIO_2%
23. ↓ PaO_2 and sat, ↑ $PaCO_2$, ↑ gradient
24. Cyanotic patient, normal PaO_2, ↓ sat
25. Non-cyanotic patient with ↓ PaO_2 and blood gas sat, normal pulse ox
26. Lactic acidosis, normal PaO_2 and pulse ox

27. Which of the following situations lowers a patient's arterial pO_2?
    a) An abnormal Hgb with an increased affinity for O_2.
    b) Anemia
    c) Carbon monoxide poisoning
    d) Lung disease with an intra-pulmonary shunt

28. A patient is admitted to the ICU with the following lab values: pH 7.40, pCO_2 38, pO_2 72, HCO_3 24. Her electrolytes are: Na 149, K 3.8, Cl 100, CO_2 24, BUN 90, and creatinine 5.3. What is/are her acid base disorder(s) ?
    a) There is no acid base disorder. She is simply hypoxic.
    b) Respiratory acidosis with a metabolic alkalosis
    c) Metabolic alkalosis and metabolic acidosis
    d) Respiratory acidosis with a concealed metabolic acidosis

29. Which of the following statements incorrectly describes carbon monoxide?
    a) It shifts the oxygen dissociation curve to the left.
    b) It lowers the PaO_2.
    c) It lowers the arterial oxygen content.
    d) It is always elevated in the blood of cigarette smokers.

30. Given the following set of electrolytes alone, calculate both the anion gap and the bicarbonate gap, then state the most likely acid-base disorder(s):
    Na 153, K 4.0, Cl 100, CO_2 23.
    a) Metabolic acidosis and metabolic alkalosis
    b) Metabolic acidosis alone
    c) Metabolic alkalosis
    d) Chronic respiratory alkalosis
    e) Must have ABG to determine if there is an acid-base disorder.

31. Which of the following most closely resembles the normal changes with aging?
    a) The alveolar-arterial pO_2 difference decreases; the pCO_2 decreases.
    b) The alveolar-arterial pO_2 difference increases; the pCO_2 decreases.
    c) The alveolar-arterial pO_2 difference increases; the pCO_2 stays the same.
    d) The alveolar-arterial pO_2 difference increases; the pCO_2 increases.

32. Which of the following conditions would be expected to derive the LEAST benefit from hyperbaric oxygen therapy?
    a) Methemoglobin toxicity
    b) Severe respiratory acidosis
    c) Cyanide poisoning
    d) Decompression sickness

33. Which of the following statements is the most accurate regarding blood gases in pulmonary embolus?
    a) They are highly variable in PE and need not be obtained as long as the sat% is adequate.
    b) 5-10% of patients with PE will have a normal A-a gradient.
    c) A normal PaO_2 essentially rules out the diagnosis of PE.
    d) A normal A-a gradient essentially rules out the diagnosis of PE.

34. The 'delta gap' or 'bicarbonate gap' is the difference between the change in anion gap and the change in serum CO_2. Which of the following very useful formulas can be used to quickly assess whether or not there is indeed such a gap, which would in turn point to a concealed metabolic alkalosis or acidosis?
    a) Na-CO_2 + 13
    b) Na-Cl + 15
    c) Na-Cl-39
    d) Na-CO_2 + anion gap
    e) Na + CO_2 - anion gap

35. A 27 yo male presents in acute respiratory failure following a serious motor vehicle accident. He is placed on assist control mechanical ventilation with an FIO_2 of 80%, a backup rate of 20, a Tidal Volume of 800cc, and no PEEP. The first gas on these settings comes back and shows good ventilation, but the pO_2 is 310 and the saturation is 100%. What is the appropriate adjustment that needs to be made in his ventilator settings?

a) Reduce the FIO_2 to 27%
b) Reduce the FIO_2 to 44%
c) Reduce the FIO_2 to 50%
d) Reduce the FIO_2 to 65%

36. Which of the following factors would not change if a climber were to ascend Mt. Everest without supplemental oxygen?

a) Barometric pressure
b) FIO_2
c) The climber's $PaCO_2$
d) The climber's PaO_2
e) The climber's pH

37. Which of the following conditions, on its own, does not lead to a metabolic alkalosis?

a) Acetazolamide therapy
b) Ethylene glycol poisoning
c) Hepatic encephalopathy
d) Renal tubular acidosis
e) Severe diarrhea

For # 38 and # 39, there may be more than one correct answer. Choose all correct answers.

38. Which of the following sets of values would be helpful in assessing the acid-base state of a patient?

a) $PaCO_2$ and HCO_3-
b) $PaCO_2$ and PaO_2
c) pH and $PaCO_2$
d) pH and PaO_2
e) pH and SaO_2

39. True statements about non-invasive blood gas monitoring include:
   a) End-tidal PCO_2 can be used to determine restoration of circulation during cardiopulmonary resuscitation.
   b) In the hemodynamically-stable patient, the pulse oximeter is equal in accuracy to the co-oximeter.
   c) In the presence of excess carboxyhemoglobin, the pulse oximeter will give a falsely high reading of oxygen saturation.
   d) The end-tidal PCO_2 is usually equal to or higher than a simultaneously-measured PCO_2.
   e) The pulse oximeter requires a detectable pulse in order to measure oxygen saturation

40. What is/are the acid-base disturbances for a patient with the following blood gas: pH 7.56, $PaCO_2$ 31, HCO_3 27, PaO_2 56 ?
   a) Acute respiratory alkalosis
   b) Chronic respiratory alkalosis
   c) Respiratory alkalosis and metabolic alkalosis
   d) Respiratory alkalosis and metabolic acidosis

41. A 59 yo woman is admitted to the ICU with shortness of breath. Her ABGs on room air and then on 6L/min are shown below:

Room Air	***6L/min***
pH 7.42	7.42
$PaCO_2$ 34	$PaCO_2$ 34
PaO_2 59	PaO_2 118
HCO_3 23	HCO_3 23
SaO_2 85	SaO_2 99

Which of the following is not included in the differential?
   a) ASD with a right-to-left shunt
   b) Mild asthma
   c) Pneumonitis
   d) Pulmonary embolus

42. A 65 yo man presents for an elective triple bypass surgery. Intraoperatively he does fine, but following extubation postoperatively he is cyanotic with mental status changes. He is reintubated at an FIO_2 of 80%. Subsequent ABG reveals: pH 7.39, $PaCO_2$ 41, PaO_2 50, HCO_3- 25. All of the following may included in the differential diagnosis except:
   a) Congestive heart failure secondary to overly aggressive hydration
   b) Mucus plugging
   c) Narcotic overdose with secondary hypoventilation
   d) Poor placement of the endotracheal tube

43. A 37 yo woman with hyperemesis gravidarum is admitted and has an nasogastric tube placed to suction. Her ABG subsequently reveals: pH 7.58, $PaCO_2$ 58, and PaO_2 98. Her electrolytes show: Na 139, Cl 73, K 2.8, HCO_3 56. What is the most likely cause for her hypercapnia?

a) Respiratory muscle weakness secondary to severe hypophosphatemia
b) COPD with respiratory failure
c) Metabolic alkalosis with appropriate compensation
d) Tracheal stenosis

44. A 33 yo fireman presents to the ER after significant smoke exposure while rescuing 3 children. His lab values on arrival show: pH 7.27, $PaCO_2$ 25, PaO_2 110, SaO_2 98, Na 138, K 5.4, Cl 101, and HCO_3 9. All of the following are correct statements except:

a) The patient has lactic acidosis.
b) Carboxyhemoglobinemia is the most likely cause of this acid-base disorder.
c) The patient should be treated with oxygen therapy immediately.
d) The patient requires treatment with sodium bicarbonate.

STATISTICS QUESTIONS

1. At a major teaching hospital, the department of epidemiology, in conjunction with the department of cardiology, conducts a study on the new model of transesophageal echocardiogram that is out. You are the statistician. The budget committee wants you to assess the negative predictive value of this new machine in their population, where the prevalence of infective endocarditis is said to be 10% among those who are tested, before procuring a number of them for their affiliated hospitals. The test has been shown to have a sensitivity of 80% and a specificity of 95%. What is the negative predictive value of this new type of TEE?
   a) 82%
   b) 79%
   c) 95%
   d) 55%

2. Six months later that same institution wins a large grant to evaluate the usefulness of a new model of PET scanner in the diagnosis of early-onset Alzheimer's disease cases, and they ask you to assess its positive predictive value in the population being studied. It is already known that the sensitivity is 68% and the specificity is 96%. Among those screened with this new technique, the prevalence of early-onset Alzheimers is 25%. What is the positive predictive value?
   a) 57%
   b) 65%
   c) 77%
   d) 85%

ANSWER KEY *

HEME

1. D
2. D
3. C
4. C
5. D
6. C
7. C
8. B
9. B
10. B
11. D
12. D
13. D
14. B
15. C
16. A
17. A
18. B
19. C
20. A
21. C
22. C
23. B
24. B
25. B
26. A
27. B
28. A
29. C
30. A
31. D
32. A
33. C
34. B
35. D
36. B
37. C
38. E
39. A
40. C
41. B
42. A
43. D
44. D

ONC

1. B
2. C
3. A
4. E
5. D
6. B
7. D
8. D
9. A
10. B
11. B
12. C
13. C
14. C
15. A
16. A
17. C
18. D
19. B
20. A
21. A
22. B
23. A
24. B
25. C

RHEUM

1. E
2. B
3. B
4. A
5. A
6. B
7. C
8. A
9. B
10. D
11. I
12. D
13. C
14. F
15. H
16. E
17. A
18. B
19. G
20. C
21. B
22. C
23. A
24. A
25. D
26. C
27. B
28. A
29. A
30. A
31. C
32. D
33. A
34. C
35. C
36. C
37. A
38. C
39. D
40. D
41. A
42. C
43. B
44. C
45. B
46. D
47. D
48. B
49. C
50. B
51. A
52. C
53. D
54. E
55. F
56. A
57. B
58. E
59. C
60. D
61. A
62. A
63. C
64. C
65. C
66. D
67. D
68. B
69. A
70. B
71. D
72. D
73. A
74. C
75. B
76. D
77. D
78. B
79. B
80. A
81. D
82. D
83. C
84. F
85. E
86. D
87. B
88. C
89. A
90. G
91. H
92. D
93. B
94. A
95. C
96. A
97. B
98. B
99. A
100.A
101.C
102.A
103.D
104.B
105.B
106.D
107.C
108.A
109.A
110.D
111.B
112.C
113.B

GI

1. A
2. E
3. C
4. B
5. D
6. C
7. D
8. B
9. C
10. A
11. C
12. A
13. A
14. B
15. D
16. B
17. B
18. A
19. B
20. D
21. B
22. D
23. A
24. B
25. D
26. C
27. A
28. C
29. D
30. E
31. G
32. C
33. F
34. A
35. B
36. A
37. A
38. C
39. A
40. D
41. C
42. D
43. D
44. E
45. C
46. B
47. A
48. E
49. B
50. F
51. C
52. A
53. D
54. A
55. C
56. B
57. A
58. C
59. A
60. C
61. B
62. D
63. B
64. C
65. C
66. B
67. A
68. B
69. A
70. A
71. B
72. A
73. B
74. A
75. B
76. A
77. C
78. K
79. J
80. F
81. I
82. L
83. B
84. G
85. A
86. E
87. H
88. D
89. D
90. B
91. C
92. B
93. C
94. B
95. B
96. C
97. B
98. C
99. A
100.C
101.D
102.A
103.E
104.F
105.G
106.H
107.B
108.C
109.C
110.A
111.D
112.D
113.B
114.C
115.D
116.A
117.B
118.C
119.B
120.C
121.C
122.A
123.B
124.A
125.B
126.B
127.A
128.A
129.B
130.C
131.B
132.A
133.B
134.D
135.C
136.C
137.B
138.A
139.C
140.C
141.A

I.D.

1. D
2. C
3. D
4. C
5. B
6. D
7. B
8. D
9. D
10. B
11. A
12. C
13. C
14. A
15. C
16. A
17. C
18. B
19. A
20. B
21. B
22. B
23. A
24. B
25. A
26. D
27. I
28. B
29. F
30. H
31. J
32. E
33. G
34. I
35. C
36. C
37. A
38. B
39. C
40. A
41. C
42. B
43. B
44. A
45. B
46. C

* *Note: Explanations accompany all answers in bold.*

ANSWER KEY *

47. B
48. D
49. C
50. B
51. A
52. B
53. A
54. B
55. C
56. D
57. E
58. A
59. C
60. D
61. B
62. A
63. A
64. B
65. B
66. C
67. C
68. B
69. C
70. A
71. B
72. B
73. C
74. D
75. C
76. D
77. A
78. B
79. A
80. C
81. E
82. B
83. E
84. D
85. D
86. E
87. D
88. C
89. A
90. E
91. D
92. D
93. D
94. D
95. A
96. D
97. B
98. A
99. A
100.C
101.F
102.G
103.B
104.E
105.D
106.H
107.C
108.C
109.G
110.A
111.C
112.B
113.A
114.B
115.C
116.D
117.E
118.A
119.D
120.C
121.A
122.B
123.A
124.D
125.F
126.A
127.C
128.B
129.C
130.C
131.D
132.B
133.B
134.A
135.C
136.A
137.B

DERM

1. A
2. F
3. D
4. G
5. C
6. B
7. I
8. E
9. H
10. D
11. F
12. E
13. B
14. G
15. A
16. H
17. I
18. C
19. D
20. C
21. B
22. A
23. C
24. J
25. K
26. A
27. F
28. I
29. D
30. G
31. L
32. B
33. H
34. E
35. A
36. D
37. I
38. D
39. B
40. H
41. F
42. G
43. A
44. B
45. C
46. E
47. J
48. H
49. K
50. C
51. A
52. C
53. B
54. C
55. A
56. C
57. B
58. C
59. B
60. B
61. F
62. B
63. C
64. A
65. E
66. G
67. D
68. E
69. F
70. B
71. C
72. A
73. D
74. D
75. A
76. B
77. C
78. B
79. B
80. D
81. C
82. C
83. A
84. B
85. A
86. C
87. A
88. A
89. D
90. A
91. B
92. D
93. B
94. C
95. B
96. B
97. A
98. D
99. D
100.A
101.B
102.D
103.C
104.B
105.C
106.B
107.A
108.C
109.A
110.D
111.C
112.B
113.A
114.C
115.C
116.D
117.C
118.D
119.C
120.A
121.B
122.A
123.C
124.B
125.B
126.A

NEURO

1. D
2. E
3. B
4. D
5. A
6. B
7. C
8. E
9. D
10. B
11. A
12. A
13. B
14. B
15. B
16. A
17. A
18. B
19. A
20. A
21. B
22. C
23. C
24. B
25. A
26. A
27. A
28. B
29. B
30. D
31. C
32. A
33. D
34. B
35. D
36. C
37. B
38. A
39. C
40. D
41. D
42. A
43. B
44. C
45. A
46. C
47. A
48. A
49. A
50. A
51. C
52. D
53. B
54. A
55. B
56. A
57. B
58. B
59. A
60. A
61. A
62. A
63. A
64. A
65. B
66. B
67. B
68. B
69. A
70. A
71. A
72. D

GERI

1. B
2. A
3. C
4. C
5. A
6. A
7. D
8. B
9. C
10. A

ALLERGY

1. D
2. C
3. A
4. C
5. C
6. B
7. D
8. A
9. A
10. B
11. C
12. D
13. B
14. C
15. G
16. A
17. E
18. F
19. A
20. D
21. B
22. A
23. A
24. B
25. A
26. B
27. F
28. C
29. A
30. G
31. D
32. A
33. B
34. B
35. E
36. A
37. B
38. D
39. C
40. B
41. B
42. F

CARDS

1. B
2. C
3. D
4. C
5. D
6. A
7. C
8. D
9. B
10. B
11. D
12. C
13. B
14. D
15. C
16. D
17. B
18. A
19. C
20. D
21. B
22. A
23. C
24. D
25. B
26. A
27. C

* *Note: Explanations accompany all answers in bold.*

ANSWER KEY *

28. A
29. C
30. D
31. B
32. E
33. D
34. A
35. B
36. B
37. A
38. A
39. B
40. A
41. B
42. A
43. A
44. A
45. A
46. B
47. A
48. C
49. C
50. F
51. D
52. B
53. G
54. A
55. E
56. C
57. G
58. E
59. F
60. I
61. D
62. A
63. H
64. B
65. D
66. A
67. E
68. F
69. D
70. C
71. G
72. H
73. B
74. B
75. A
76. D
77. A
78. B
79. C
80. D
81. B
82. A
83. C
84. C
85. D
86. A
87. D
88. B
89. D
90. B
91. D
92. A
93. C
94. B
95. C
96. C
97. B
98. A
99. D
100.B
101.C
102.C
103.D
104.B
105.A
106.B
107.C
108.D
109.B
110.A
111.B
112.B
113.B
114.C
115.D
116.A
117.C
118.D
119.A
120.A
121.B
122.B
123.A
124.A
125.C
126.A
127.B
128.A
129.D
130.B
131.A
132.F
133.F
134.E
135.D
136.C
137.B
138.D
139.C
140.A
141.B
142.A
143.A
144.A
145.A
146.B
147.A
148.B
149.A
150.B
151.B

PULM

1. B
2. A
3. B
4. C
5. B
6. A
7. D
8. B
9. C
10. D
11. D
12. A
13. D
14. D
15. A
16. C
17. D
18. B
19. C
20. C
21. C
22. D
23. A
24. B
25. A
26. A
27. C
28. B
29. B
30. C
31. C
32. B
33. C
34. C
35. D
36. B
37. B
38. C
39. A
40. D
41. D
42. C
43. D
44. A
45. C
46. A
47. B
48. B
49. C
50. A
51. D
52. C
53. B
54. B
55. I
56. H
57. C
58. B
59. E
60. F
61. D
62. G
63. A
64. G
65. B
66. C
67. H
68. F
69. D
70. A
71. E
72. A
73. B
74. C
75. A
76. B
77. B
78. B
79. C
80. D
81. B
82. B
83. A
84. C
85. D
86. B
87. D
88. B
89. A
90. C
91. D

ENDO

1. A
2. B
3. A
4. C
5. A
6. B
7. A
8. B
9. E
10. B
11. D
12. B
13. A
14. E
15. A
16. B
17. D
18. C
19. B
20. A
21. C
22. A
23. B
24. B
25. C
26. A
27. B
28. B
29. A
30. A
31. D
32. C
33. B
34. A
35. D
36. D
37. C
38. A
39. C
40. A
41. B
42. B
43. A
44. B
45. D
46. B
47. C
48. A
49. C
50. A
51. B
52. D
53. A
54. D
55. A
56. E
57. E
58. C
59. C
60. C
61. A
62. B
63. C
64. A
65. C
66. C
67. A
68. B
69. C
70. B
71. C
72. B
73. D
74. D
75. B
76. D
77. A
78. C
79. C
80. A
81. D
82. B
83. C
84. A
85. D
86. D
87. A
88. B
89. C
90. A
91. A
92. A
93. B
94. C
95. B
96. A

RENAL

1. A
2. D
3. E
4. B
5. B
6. C
7. C
8. C
9. C
10. D
11. A
12. C
13. C
14. C
15. J
16. A,J
17. H
18. F
19. B
20. A,C,D
21. A,E,I
22. F,G
23. F,G
24. F
25. A,B,E
26. K
27. A,B
28. I
29. E
30. A
31. I
32. B
33. A
34. E
35. C
36. B
37. D
38. A
39. C
40. B
41. C
42. C
43. A
44. C
45. D
46. B
47. C
48. B
49. B
50. C
51. C
52. B
53. B
54. E
55. A
56. F
57. A
58. B
59. D
60. C
61. A
62. B
63. E
64. A
65. E

* *Note: Explanations accompany all answers in bold.*

A N S W E R K E Y

ANSWER KEY *

66. E
67. F
68. J
69. B
70. D
71. A
72. G
73. F
74. E
75. H
76. I
77. C
78. A,C
79. B
80. B
81. A,B
82. A
83. A,B,C
84. A,B,D
85. C
86. C
87. A
88. B
89. D
90. C
91. A
92. J
93. A,M
94. C
95. G
96. B,O
97. B,O
98. K
99. O,P
100.D,F
101.L
102.D
103.H
104.I
105.E
106.A
107.N,Q

TOX

1. B
2. C
3. C
4. D
5. H
6. E
7. B
8. C
9. G
10. F
11. A
12. I
13. B
14. A

ABG's

1. D
2. C
3. A
4. B
5. A
6. B
7. A
8. A
9. D
10. C
11. A
12. B
13. C
14. A
15. B
16. K
17. A
18. G
19. J
20. C
21. A
22. D
23. I
24. F
25. E
26. B
27. E
28. C
29. B
30. A
31. C
32. B
33. B
34. C
35. C
36. B
37. C
38. A,C
39. A,C,E
40. C
41. A
42. C
43. C
44. D

STATS

1. C
2. D

** Note: Explanations accompany all answers in bold.*

HEMATOLOGY

2. Acute glomerulonephritis, ARF, DIC, HTN, Pulm HTN, HUS, TTP, PAN, SLE, HELLP syndrome, and preeclampsia all can lead to microangiopathic hemolytic anemia, a Coombs negative anemia. Therefore, *all* of these can produce schistocytes.

3. The Philadelphia chromosome does indeed result in the formation of a chimeric bcr-abl gene, but this translocation results in *maturational block* among the granulocytes so that you can see all stages of granulocytes on a CML peripheral blood smear. This translocation is also responsible for blast crisis in CML.

4. The "1 to 1 dilution test" simply mixes "one part" patient serum with "one part" control serum (i.e. serum that is known to have all the factors present) and checks to see if the PT or PTT (whatever the coagulopathy) normalizes with the addition of the control serum. If there is no "correction" in the PT or PTT, then that means that there was in fact no factor deficiency, and that, instead, there must a factor inhibitor present (e.g. Factor VIII inhibitor, lupus anticoagulant, anticardiolipin antibody, etc.).

5. Delayed transfusion reactions occur *3-5 days after* receiving a transfusion of packed red blood cells.

6. H.A.T.T. develops 3-15 days after initiating heparin, with a median time *of 10 days after* initiation.

7. 5-10% of PNH patients will develop *leukemia* (AML), not lymphoma.

8. The typical order of events in vitamin B12 deficiency is: 1st) ↑ in serum homocysteine and MMA (methylmalonic acid); 2nd) Serum B12 ↓; 3rd) MCV increases but is still normal and *hypersegmented neutrophils appear; 4th) MCV ↑ beyond normal*; 5th) anemia develops; and 6th) symptoms are seen.

9. As opposed to TTP, in HUS there is *no fever*. The *classic triad* is microangiopathic hemolytic anemia, thrombocytopenia, and renal failure.

10. There is no increased risk of infections in patients with trait only.

11. Sequestration crisis indeed causes pooling of RBCs in the spleen (and is primarily seen in young children); however, it is *vaso-occlusive crisis*, also referred to as 'painful' or 'infarctive' crisis, that *causes autosplenectomy* due to intravascular obstruction and subsequent hypoxia.

18. *Bone pain* is the most common symptom in myeloma, affecting nearly 70 percent of patients.

20. The Philadelphia chromosome is simply a translocation between chromosomes 9 and 22 (t9,22) that results in a so-called chimeric bcr-abl gene that prematurely arrests granulocyte maturation.

21. *Addison*-like wasting syndrome!

22. The erythopoetin level is usually decreased.

23. Normal PT and PTT (it's just the bleeding time that is↑)

24. DIC is due to a "consumptive coagulopathy", so enough is made; it's just that the factors are quickly consumed within the microvascular thrombi that form. When these are consumed, a bleeding diathesis can ensue.

25. All routine clotting tests are normal! (including PTT)

26. Factor V Leiden deficiency or activated Protein C resistance ("aPC resistance") accounts for between 30-50% (!) of patients with "idiopathic" venous thrombosis.

35. If transfusions are needed, select non-related donors and use leukocyte-depleted PRBCs and single-donor platelets. Family members should not be transfusion donors since they are more likely to sensitize the patient to minor HLA antigens present in the donor, but absent in the patient.

36. High dose gamma globulin works by *blocking* the phagocytic cell Fc receptors *and is used in emergencies only.*

37. Hemochromatosis is caused by inappropriate increase in intestinal iron absorption.

39. Factor VII is part of the extrinsic pathway!

ONCOLOGY

1. A primary tumor size exceeding 2.5 cm is formally considered a poor prognosticator.

3. Remember, based on Duke's criteria, colorectal carcinomas that extend thru the serosa are B2 and require the addition of chemotherapy.

4. Hypercalcemia is a paraneoplastic phenomenon associated with squamous cell carcinoma, *not* small cell. This is felt to be due to a PTH-related protein, or PTHrP.

5. Remember, because small cell lung ca has usually spread by the time of diagnosis, surgery is not appropriate, but is instead reserved for early stage (I-IIIA) non-small cell lung carcinoma. Limited small cell carcinoma is managed with chemotherapy and radiation.

6. Remember, preoperative pulmonary workup for lung carcinoma is done as follows: if preoperative $FEV_1 < 2L$, MVV < 50% or DL_{CO} < 60%, the patient requires a quantitative V/Q scan to assess the *expected post-op* FEV_1*, which must be > 1.3L.*

7. This is a common "trick question". It's actually just an exception that you have to know. Early Hodgkin's Lymphoma (I-IIIA) gets radiation alone, unless there's bulky disease. If there's bulky disease, it doesn't matter what the actual stage: the patient must also receive chemotherapy.

9. Low grade NHLs include multiple myeloma, Waldenstrom's macroglobulinemia, and CLL. DLCL (diffuse large cell lymphoma) is the important NHL that is classified as "intermediate grade". High grades include lymphoblastic lymphoma and small non-cleaved lymphomas. Small non-cleaved lymphomas are further divided into Burkitt's and Non-Burkitt's lymphomas.

10. Size cutoff is 6mm, roughly the size of a pencil-head eraser.

12. Answer c should read "before age 50"!

19-20. The Philadelphia chromosome is present in CML, and absent in CLL. While platelets are normal or reduced in CLL, depending on the stage, the platelets in CML can be normal, reduced, *or* elevated.

25. Hyperphosphatemia, which can be caused by the release of intracellular phosphate pools by tumor cell lysis, produces a reciprocal depression in serum calcium, which causes severe neuromuscular irritability and tetany. Deposition of calcium phosphate in the kidney and hyperphosphatemia may cause renal failure. Potassium is the principal intracellular cation, and massive destruction of malignant cells may lead to hyperkalemia. Hyperkalemia in patients with renal failure may rapidly become life-threatening.

RHEUMATOLOGY

10. While indeed episcleritis and uveitis are extra-articular manifestations of RA, keratoconjunctivitis sicca, from secondary Sjögren's, is the #1 opthalmic complication. In fact, fifteen to twenty percent of persons with RA may develop Sjögren's syndrome with attendant keratoconjunctivitis sicca.

20. Another difference between these two rheumatologic conditions is that Still's disease is *seronegative* and Felty's is *seropositive.*

34. HLA-DR4, *not* 3

35. Staph aureus and Salmonella, *not* streptococcus in sickle cell

37. It's *nephrolithiasis*, not cholelithiasis! → Half of patients with uric acid stones have *gout*.

39. Allopurinol can cause eosinophilia; leukopenia; leukocytosis; *thrombocytopenia*; agranulocytosis; sore throat; anemia; and aplastic anemia;

45. *HypOphosphatemia!* Also→*hypomagnesemia*

46. *HLA-B12 and HLA-B5* are associated with Behçet's, not B27

47. In DISH, there's a sensation of stiffness, yet *relatively well-preserved spinal motion*

48. *Straightening of the lumbar spine*. In the lumbar spine, progression of the disease leads to straightening, caused by loss of lordosis, and reactive sclerosis, caused by osteitis of the anterior corners of the vertebral bodies with subsequent erosion, leading to "squaring" of the vertebral bodies

49. The term is "*keratoderma blenorrhagicum*"!!

56. The spondylitis/sacroiliitis indeed occur in ~5% of IBD patients, indeed may predate the onset of bowel symptoms, but are independent of bowel disease activity, and so are unaffected by colectomy. This is in *contrast* to the peripheral arthritis of IBD.

57. Patients with IBD alone *do not* have an increased incidence of HLA-B27 nor do they have an increased risk of developing spondylitis.

59. It's *asymmetric*!

60. Responds *well* to therapy. And that combination of antibiotics I mentioned is, in fact, *recommended* (*NOT*: "may be tried")

61. The joint appearance and presentation is generally similar to *rheumatoid arthritis*.

62. Thyrotoxicosis is a cause of clubbing.

63. *Inclusion body myositis responds poorly to steroids*! *Poikiloderma* is a term used to describe a patch of skin with (1) reticulated hypo- and hyperpigmentation, (2) wrinkling secondary to epidermal atrophy, and (3) telangiectasias. Poikiloderma does not imply a single disease entity. It is seen in skin damaged by ionizing radiation, in the disorders poikiloderma vasculare atrophicans (PVA) and xeroderma pigmentosum, as well as in patients with connective-tissue diseases, primarily dermatomyositis (DM).

78. Anti-Smith is the most specific autoantibody for SLE, even more than anti-ds DNA. The World Health Organization categorizes lupus nephritis into six histologic classes. *Class I* consists of a normal biopsy on light microscopy with occasional mesangial deposits on immunofluorescence microscopy. Patients in this category usually do not have clinical renal disease. Patients with *class II* or mesangial lupus nephritis have prominent mesangial deposits of IgG, IgM, and C3 on immunofluorescence and electron microscopy. Mesangial lupus nephritis is designated as class IIA when the glomeruli are normal by light microscopy and class IIB when there is mesangial hypercellularity. Microscopic hematuria is common with this lesion, and 25 to 50 percent of patients have moderate proteinuria. Nephrotic syndrome is not seen, and renal survival is excellent (>90 percent at 5 years). *Class III* describes focal segmental proliferative lupus nephritis with necrosis or sclerosis affecting fewer than 50 percent of glomeruli. Up to one-third of patients have nephrotic syndrome, and glomerular filtration is impaired in 15 to 25 percent. In *class IV* or diffuse proliferative lupus nephritis, most glomeruli show cell proliferation, often with crescent formation. Other features on light microscopy include fibrinoid necrosis and "wire loops," which are caused by basement membrane thickening and mesangial interposition between basement membrane and endothelial cells. Deposits of IgG, IgM, IgA, and C3 are evident by immunofluorescence, and crescents stain positive for fibrin. Electron microscopy reveals numerous immune deposits in mesangial, subepithelial, and subendothelial locations. Tubuloreticular structures are frequently seen in endothelial cells. These are not specific for lupus nephritis and are also seen in human immunodeficiency virus (HIV)-associated nephropathy. Electron microscopy may also reveal curvilinear parallel arrays of microfibrils, measuring approximately 10 to 15 nm in diameter, with "thumbprinting," similar to those seen in cryoglobulinemia. Nephrotic syndrome and renal insufficiency are present in at least 50 percent of patients with class IV disease. Diffuse proliferative lupus nephritis is the most aggressive renal lesion in SLE, and as many as 30 percent of these patients progress to terminal renal failure. *Class V* is termed membranous lupus nephritis because of its similarity to idiopathic membranous glomerulopathy. Thickening of the GBM is evident by light microscopy. Electron microscopy reveals predominant subepithelial deposits in addition to subendothelial and mesangial deposits.

Proliferative changes may also be evident, but the predominant pattern is that of membranous glomerulopathy. Most patients present with nephrotic syndrome (90 percent), but significant impairment of GFR is relatively unusual (10 percent). Tubulointerstitial changes such as active infiltration by inflammatory cells, tubular atrophy, and interstitial fibrosis are seen to varying degrees in lupus nephritis and are most severe in classes III and IV, especially in patients with long-standing disease. *Class VI* probably represents the end stages of proliferative lupus nephritis and is characterized by diffuse glomerulosclerosis and advanced tubulointerstitial disease. These patients are often hypertensive, may have nephrotic syndrome, and usually have impaired GFR.

93. Beta blockers are <u>*contraindicated*</u> since they will ↑ the spasm.

94. *Thromboangiitis obliterans is the pathophysiology* in Buerger's disease and can lead to ulcers of the distal upper extremity as well as the lower extremity. Buerger's disease occurs primarily in young men (ages 25 to 40) who smoke or have been smokers.

101. Both are estrogenic on bone. Both are antiestrogenic on breast and CNS. However, raloxifene is antiestrogenic and tamoxifen is estrogenic vs. the endometrium.

102. <u>*Hyper*</u>thyroidism.

104. Phosphorous is ↓.

105. CHRONIC renal failure→2° hyperparathyroidism→renal osteodystrophy with a syndrome of osteitis fibrosa cystica, osteomalacia, and hyperparathyroidism

107. Sacrum, spine, femur, tibia, skull, and pelvis

108. Nonrestorative sleep or awakening unrefreshed has been observed in most patients with fibromyalgia. Sleep electroencephalographic studies in patients with fibromyalgia have shown disruption of normal stage 4 sleep [non-rapid eye movement (NREM) sleep] by many repeated alpha-wave intrusions. The idea that stage 4 sleep deprivation has a role in causing this disorder was supported by the observation that symptoms of fibromyalgia developed in normal subjects whose stage 4 sleep was disrupted artificially by induced alpha-wave intrusions. This sleep disturbance, however, has been demonstrated in healthy individuals, in emotionally distressed individuals, and in patients with sleep apnea, fever, osteoarthritis, or rheumatoid arthritis.

109. *HYPERgammaglobulinemia can be seen. Other labs that can be seen: ↑ESR, anemia of chronic disease, p-ANCA, hypereosinophilia*; the leukocyte count is elevated with a predominance of neutrophils; Hep B surface antigen in some patients

110. *TYPE I is monoclonal; TYPES II AND III are polyclonal* primarily. Cryoglobulins are immunoglobulins that precipitate in the cold and can be composed of either monoclonal immunoglobulin, usually generated by a lymphoproliferative malignancy (type I); a mixture of polyclonal immunoglobulin (usually IgG) and monoclonal immunoglobulin (usually IgM) directed to epitopes on polyclonal IgG (type II); or a mixture of polyclonal antibodies, one or more having anti-IgG activity (type III).

111. The vasculitis affects arterioles, capillaries, and veinules and does not discriminate.

112. Intraluminal thrombus-containing microabscesses of the vessels is likely the primary event, and so Buerger's is certainly NOT considered a true classic vasculitis.

GASTROENTEROLOGY

3. Hepatitis D can occur as a 'superinfection' in patients with underlying chronic HBV or as a 'coinfection' during acute HBV infection. Superinfection, therefore, implies a chronic process. Nevertheless, HDV in this setting may have an acute worsening of liver disease and a more rapid progression to cirrhosis with secondary/increased ascites. Alcoholic cardiomyopathy, a dilated cardiomyopathy, will *not* present acutely as such.

4. Remember, one of the key features of IBS is that it does *not* awaken the patient.

5. Chronic hepatitis is defined by an elevation in transaminases for at least *six months*.

6. Because some HCV-infected patients may be only intermittently HCV RNA +, a single negative test cannot be used to R/O chronic infection, and repeat testing at 3-6 mo intervals by PCR is indicated to check for *chronic infection with intermittent viremia*.

12. HDV can occur as a superinfection in patients with underlying <u>*chronic*</u> Hep B or as a coinfection during <u>*acute*</u> HBV infection.

13. Over 85% of the time (*not* 15-20%)

14. Advise patients not to share razors and toothbrushes. Covering an open wound is recommended. However, it is **not** recommended to avoid close contact with family members or to avoid sharing meals or utensils.

15. *Membranoproliferative* GN!

16. Resembles hepatitis **A** epidemiologically, as it is also enterically transmitted.

17. Indeed young women, primarily; however, average age is *10-20 yo*, not 20-30.

18. PBC is an idiopathic disease of middle-aged women affecting the *small* bile ducts. Common symptoms include pruritis and steatorrhea (2° to progressive cholestasis).

19. *Indeed,* ulcerative colitis is associated in 70% of cases. *However*, it may come *before, during, or after* the PSC.

21. Vinyl chloride causes ANGIOSARCOMA, not peliosis hepatis. Incidentally, thoratrast and anabolic steroids also may lead to angiosarcoma

23. CUSHING'S syndrome (↑cortisol) NOT ADDISON'S!!!!!!

24. In scleroderma manometry reveals decreased amplitude or disappearance of peristaltic waves in the lower two-thirds of the esophagus. Also the resting pressure of the LES is subnormal, but sphincter relaxation is normal.

26. Remember, it's Shigella, *not salmonella*, that causes bloody diarrhea!

27. In scleroderma, one can see:
    - Roentgenographic features of the second and third portions of the duodenum and of the jejunum include **dilatation**, loss of the usual feathery pattern, and delayed disappearance of barium.
    - Hypomotility of the small intestine produces symptoms of bloating and abdominal pain and may suggest an intestinal obstruction or paralytic **ileus** (pseudoobstruction);
    - Motility studies show aperistalsis in the body of the esophagus; LES incompetence can lead to severe reflux

28. If a patient with frank neurologic or psychiatric disease does not have Kayser-Fleischer rings when examined by a trained observer using a slit lamp, the diagnosis of Wilson's disease can be excluded. Zinc salts are effective at doses of 150 mg/d of elemental zinc in patients whose copper stores have been reduced by penicillamine or trientine. Zinc must *not*, however, be given together with penicillamine or trientine since zinc can chelate either drug and form complexes that are ineffective.

36. Response Of Complications Of Ulcerative Colitis To Colectomy
    - ***Positive Response***
        - **P** eripheral arthropathy (don't confuse with hemochromatosis, where treatment *does not* improve the arthropathy)
        - **P** yoderma gangrenosum (and the other dermatologic manifestation, erythema nodosum)
        - **P** ara-rectal disease

    - ***Unresponsive***
        - **S** pondilitis, Ankylosing (Remember, 'S' for Stays the same!)
        - **S** clerosing cholangitis (Remember, 'S' for Stays the same!)

37. Hyp**ER**calcemia (± MEN I)
    - Somatostatin is the drug of choice for symptom control.

38. The diarrhea in glucagonoma is **not** steatorrheic. *Additional findings include*:
    - ***Necrolytic migratory erythema***: a transient bullous or crusting rash, often involving perineum and leaving residual pigmentation
    - ***Glucose intolerance:*** remember, glucagon mobilizes glucose stores.
    - ↓cholesterol; spontaneous, asymptomatic remissions common.
    - Tx: somatostatin for the diarrhea, anticoagulants for any thromboses, insulin if required.

39. If resection is curative, patients can expect a normal life expectancy. If not, average life expectancy is only 2 years.

40. The secretin test can confirm the diagnosis by demonstrating a *paradoxical* ↑ (not "exaggerated ↓") in gastrin level in response to infused secretin. In patients who have simple PUD, secretin acts to inhibit gastrin, since it inhibits gastrin normally. In ZES, though, it's opposite!

41. Remember, BP drops 2° to vasodilatation from the release of vasoactive mediators. This causes a compensatory ↑ in pulse.

42. 90% of the primary tumors are found in the *terminal ileum.*

55. Patients with **gluten**-sensitive enteropathy are at risk of developing *intestinal T cell lymphomas*. They involve the ileum predominantly. These diseases present with abdominal pain, obstruction, and perforation, and surgical debulking is often indicated in their management. Intestinal lymphoma 2° to celiac sprue should be suspected in patients with malabsorption with the following findings: (1) a malabsorption syndrome in which clinical and biopsy features resemble those of celiac sprue but in which there is an incomplete response to a **gluten**-free diet, (2) the presence of *abdominal pain* and *fever*, and (3) signs and symptoms of intestinal obstruction. The usual stigmata of generalized **lymphoma** are frequently absent.

56. MEGALOBLASTIC anemia (not microcytic) is seen as bacteria consume B12. Interestingly, ↓B12 may also be 2° to loss of intrinsic factor that occurs with gastrectomy. Blind loop syndrome is also known as "stagnant" loop syndrome.

57. The purpose of the D-Xylose test is to show if the source of malabsorption is pancreatic insufficiency or small intestine! If the D-Xylose is abnormal, the small intestine is the culprit. THEN you must differentiate between mucosal vs. bacterial overgrowth etiologies by a number of ways. Jejunal aspirates and small bowel biopsy may reveal a mucosal lesion. ^{14}C-xylose/glucose/lactulose breath tests (measure exhaled $14CO_2$) and Schilling tests (checks for B12 malabsorption) may reveal bacterial overgrowth.

58. The secretin test is diagnostic of pancreatic exocrine insufficiency if there is a DECREASE in pancreatic fluid output and bicarbonate secretion after an IV dose of secretin. This test is performed under fluoroscopic guidance.

59. *At time of admission or diagnosis:*
    1. Age >55yo
    2. WBC >16
    3. Glucose (serum) >200
    4. **LDH >350**
    5. SGOT (AST) >250

60. *During initial 48 hours*

1. **↓ in Hct >10%**
2. Serum Ca <8
3. ↑ in BUN >5
4. Arterial pO_2<60
5. Base deficit >4
6. Estimated fluid sequestration >600 cc

61. Pseudocysts are indeed fluid collections. However, most of the time they resolve **SPONTANEOUSLY** within a few weeks.

62. *DRUGS THAT CAUSE PANCREATITIS: "PD FAST VET"...*
(as in "Pretty Fast corVETte")

P entamidine
D di (didanosine)
F urosemide
A zathioprine
S ulfa
T hiazides
V alproic acid
E strogen
T etracycline

63. Although the gallbladder is usually enlarged in patients with carcinoma of the head of the pancreas, it is palpable in less than 50 percent of cases (**Courvoisier**'s **sign**). However, the presence of an enlarged gallbladder in a jaundiced patient without biliary colic should suggest malignant obstruction of the extrahepatic biliary tree. Trousseau's sign is simply recurrent migratory thrombophlebitis secondary to pancreatic ca. "Double-duct" sign is obstruction, and therefore visible dilatation, of both bile and pancreatic ducts, and is secondary to pancreatic ca; a classic presentation.

In **ACUTE** pancreatitis the most frequent abnormalities include (1) a localized ileus, usually involving the jejunum ("**sentinel loop**"); (2) a generalized ileus with air-fluid levels; (3) the "colon cutoff sign," which results from isolated distention of the transverse colon; (4) duodenal distention with air-fluid levels; and (5) a mass, which is frequently a pseudocyst. In **CHRONIC** pancreatitis, an important radiographic finding is pancreatic calcification.

64. May lead to intestinal *lymphangiectasia*, and indeed can cause hyperpigmentation, heart failure, endocarditis, and uveitis. More commonly see diarrhea, fever, LN, migratory arthralgias and neurologic symptoms.

71. The ^{13}C and ^{14}C UBTs **can also be used to confirm eradication after treatment** (as well as to detect active H. Pylori infection). Stool testing is another noninvasive method shown to compare well with the breath test. However, with the urease breath test, ***proper timing is important***: testing must be done ≥ 2 weeks after cessation of maintenance antisecretory therapy and ≥ 4 weeks after completion of antibiotic therapy (4 weeks post treatment for stool antigen detection). Remember, **antibody testing with ELISA** is less useful in the evaluation of posttreatment response because high levels of antibodies to H. pylori remain for variable and extended periods. However, for an individual more than a year out from therapy, seroconversion is a reliable indicator of successful eradication. The CLO test is an agar test that turns color when presented with H. Pylori in a biopsy specimen obtained during endoscopy.

89. Acute colitis may be caused by a variety of infectious agents. Often presenting with bloody diarrhea, infectious colitis may be difficult to distinguish from IBD at initial presentation, and severe cases may present with colonic dilation mimicking toxic megacolon. In addition, an unexplained exacerbation of IBD symptoms may be due to a superimposed infectious colitis. Campylobacter jejuni is also one of the agents that can trigger an HLA-B27 positive reactive arthritis.

91-98. Fibrosis is more common in Crohn's; rectal bleeding, toxic megacolon and malignant potential are more common in UC.

100. Among the extraintestinal manifestations: ***the severity of joint and skin disease mirrors the severity of colitis.*** On the other hand, ankylosing spondylitis and sacroiliitis ***DO NOT*** mirror the colitis.

109. Angiography is **not** helpful in the management of patients with presumed ischemic colitis because a remediable occlusive lesion is very rarely found.

110. Meig's is transudate. Rather than the total protein content of ascites, some authors prefer the use of a *serum-ascites albumin gradient* (SAG) to characterize ascites. The gradient correlates directly with portal pressure. A gradient >1.1 g/dL is characteristic of uncomplicated cirrhotic ascites; a gradient <1.1 g/dL is seen in conditions characterized by exudative ascites, as with all the other choices given.

111. An ascitic fluid total leukocyte count of greater than 500 cells/uL (with a proportion of polymorphonuclear leukocytes of 50 percent or greater) or ascitic PMN count >250 cells/uL should suggest the diagnosis of SBP.

112. Worsening azotemia, hypOnatremia, progressive oliguria, and hypOtension are the hallmarks of the hepatorenal syndrome.

117. There is in fact a risk of malignant transformation from hamartomas that is *present, though quite low.*

139. Leukopenia , though only occasionally seen, is considered and extrahepatic feature of autoimmune hepatitis.

140. Remember, in Wilson's disease the ceruloplasmin is *depressed*, as is the ***total*** serum copper. The ***free*** serum copper is *elevated*, as is the urine and liver copper.

INFECTIOUS DISEASE

1. The West Nile-like virus cannot be spread directly from person to person and there is no evidence that a person can get the virus from handling an infected bird.

2. Indeed EBNA IgG does indicate prior infection, but it persists lifelong.

3. Patients who have never had chicken pox can get chicken pox by exposure to someone with shingles (*but can't get zoster* since to contract zoster you have to have had chicken pox, as zoster is a manifestation of reactivation of a previous infection).

4. The polyarthropathy of Parvovirus B19 is *symmetric.*

5. Rotavirus in a watery diarrheal illness of children seen primarily in the winter and is frequently contracted through swimming pools.

6. **HPV** is associated with *oral leukoplakia*, which is NOT the same thing as oral *hairy* leukoplakia, which is associated with **EBV**.

7. HRIG + vaccine are indeed useful, but only if begun *prior to the onset of symptoms.*

8. If a pregnant woman is non-immune and is rechecked 2-3 weeks later and has seroconverted, a *therapeutic abortion* should be considered.

13. Triple therapy optimally refers to two nucleoside analogues (one group A drug and one group B drug) plus one drug from *either* the non- nucleoside analogues or from the protease inhibitors. Adding one group 'A' drug to one group 'B' drug prevents additive toxicities.

15. *Rifampin* should not be administered concurrently with **protease inhibitors or non**nucleoside reverse transcriptase inhibitors. Rifabutin is an alternative. Even then, *rifabutin* should not be given with saquinivir or delavirdine.

16. Glucocorticoids are indicated for use in the treatment of any patient with HIV infection and PCP in whom the PaO_2 is under 70 mmHg or in whom the a-A gradient is over 35 mmHg. In this setting, several clinical trials have shown clear benefit from glucocorticoids, with approximately a 50 percent decrease in mortality (from 40 to 20 percent) and a 50 percent decrease in the number of patients requiring mechanical ventilatory support. The only significant side effect has been an increased incidence of thrush. Adjunct glucocorticoid therapy should be started as soon as possible after the diagnosis is made, preferably no later than 36 to 72 h. In fact, glucocorticoids added later in the course of disease have not been shown to confer any clinical benefit and have been associated with an increased risk of other opportunistic infections. The recommended length of glucocorticoid therapy is 21 days.

17. Pseudomonas aeruginosa causes ecthyma gangrenosum in **neutropenic** patients, commonly following chemotherapy.

Q#		
18	B	↑
19	A	↓
20	B	↓
21	B	↓
22	B	↑
23	A	↓
24	B	↑
25	A	↓

38. Clinical presentation includes fever, chills, headache, **dry** cough, stiff neck.

39. Augmentin (Amoxicillin + clavulinate) is the initial drug of choice as coverage is needed against staph aureus, pasteurella multocida, capnocytophaga, and anaerobes, so that amoxicillin on its own, is a *poor* first choice.

40. CSD → immunoCOMPETENT; BA→immunoSUPPRESSED

41. Although the prevalence of listeriosis among persons infected with HIV is much **HIGHER** than that in the general population, listeriosis is a relatively **UNCOMMON** opportunistic infection in AIDS.

42. **Approximately two-thirds of patients with disseminated gonococcal infection are WOMEN.**

43. Any febrile patient with a petechial rash should be considered to have meningococcal infection. Blood for cultures should be taken immediately and **treatment begun without awaiting confirmation.**

44. *Brucella* is transmitted most commonly through the ingestion of untreated milk or milk products, raw meat, or bone marrow. However, the organism can be contracted via inhalation during contact with animals, especially by children and by slaughterhouse, farm, and laboratory workers. Other routes of infection for at-risk workers include skin abrasion, autoinoculation, and conjunctival splashing. The organism has been transmitted from person to person through the placenta, during breast feeding, and (in rare instances) during sexual activity.

45. That's erythema ***multiforme*** and the SJS.
46. Actually, actinomyces is associated with rib bone **destruction**. Actinomycotic infection of the bone is usually due to adjacent soft-tissue infection but may be

associated with trauma (e.g., fracture of the mandible) or hematogenous spread. Because of slow disease progression**, new-bone formation and bone destruction are seen concomitantly**. *However, bony destruction usually predominates.* Infection of an extremity is uncommon and is usually a result of trauma. Skin, subcutaneous tissue, muscle, and bone (with periostitis or acute or chronic osteomyelitis) are involved alone or in various combinations.

47. *Endemic* **typhus** is a <u>flea-borne</u> disease. *Epidemic* typhus is <u>louse-borne</u>. Human Granulocytic **Erlichiosis** is carried by the deer tick ixodes dammini (as is Lyme disease!) and ixodes scapularis, and Human Monocytic Erlichiosis is caused by the dog tick amblyomma americanum and dermacentor variabilis (similar to **Rocky Mountain Spotted Fever**). Rocky Mt. Spotted Fever in the Mid-Atlantic states is generally transmitted by the American **dog tick**, dermacentor variabilis. History of tick bite given in >80% of cases. **Q fever** results from infection with coxiella burnetii. Q fever is a zoonosis. The primary sources of human infection are infected cattle, sheep, and goats. In the infected female mammal, C. burnetii localizes to the uterus and the mammary glands; infection is reactivated during pregnancy, and high concentrations of C. burnetii are found in the placenta. At parturition, C. burnetii is dispersed as an aerosol, and infection follows inhalation of these organisms by a susceptible host. Infected female animals shed the organism in milk for weeks or months after parturition.

49. RMSF is ***not* seen in the Rocky Mt. States** (go figure!), but is most common in the **mid-Atlantic states (i.e. MD, VA, NC, and Georgia)**; transmitted by the American **dog tick**, Dermacentor variabilis. Moreover, a history of a tick bite is given in **> 80%** of the cases!!

50. **Laboratories show ↓WBC, ↓platelets, and ↑LFTs.**

58. Brucella is a gram-negative bacillus.

59. E. faecium is inherently penicillin-resistant.

60. Prompt antibiotic therapy ***does not*** appear to prevent the development of post-streptococcal glomerulonephritis as ***compared to*** rheumatic fever following throat infection.

61. Major and minor Jones criteria: **"S.A.F.E.R. C.A.S.E.S." ...**
(must have 2 major *or* 1 major + 2 minor criteria to make the diagnosis) **...**

Minor	**Major**
Sore throat	**C**arditis
Arthralgias	**A**SO titre↑
Fever	**S**yndenham's chorea
EKG changes;↑ ESR	**E**rythema Marginatum
Rheumatic History	**S**Q nodules

62. *Clinical manifestations usually appear 1-3 weeks after the onset of pharyngitis.*

75. TETANUS PROPHYLAXIS IN WOUND MANAGEMENT (32nd ed. Sanford Guide)

History of Tetanus Immunization	**Dirty, Tetanus-prone Wound**		**Clean Minor Wounds**	
	TD[1,2]	TIG	Td	TIG
Unknown or < 3doses*	Yes	Yes	Yes	**NO**
≥3 doses**	No[3]	No	No[4]	No

* *"YES" to all except TIG for clean minor wounds!*
** *"NO" to all !*

[1] Td = Tetanus & diptheria toxoids adsorbed (adults)
TIG = Tetanus immune globulin (human)
[2] Yes if wound > 24 hours old.
For children < 7 years. DPT (DT if pertussis vaccine contraindicated);
For persons ≥ 7 years, Td preferred to tetanus toxoid alone.
[3] Yes if > 5 years since last booster
[4] Yes if > 10 years since last booster

93-94. Most students are surprised to learn that permanent pacemakers and implantable automatic defibrillators do not require prophylaxis. Neither does routine cavity filling with a local anesthetic. Remember, with dental visits, it's essentially extractions and periodontal procedures that necessitate prophylaxis. Similarly, while rigid bronchoscopy requires prophylaxis, flexible bronchoscopy does not. And while sclerotherapy of esophageal varices and dilatation of esophageal stricture require antibiotic coverage, TEE and EGD without biopsy do not.

95. Reactive thrombocytosis from endocarditis rarely approach levels that are so critical that they cause, for example, significant sludging.

112. Ehrlichiae are small, gram-negative, obligately intracellular bacteria that grow as microcolonies in phagosomes. The appearance of the cytoplasmic inclusion, a vacuolar *cluster* of Giemsa-stained ehrlichiae in phagocytes, accounts for its name, ***morula***, the Latin word for *mulberry*. However, morula may also be seen in other diseases, such as multiple myeloma. Pappenheimer bodies, remember, are the hyposegmented neutrophils that are frequently seen post-splenectomy.

118. Patients <35 yo with epididymitis should be treated as for GC + Chlamydia since these are the 2 most common culprits in this age group. Patients > 35 yo with epididymitis should be treated for enterobacteriaceae. E. Coli is the most common culprit here, especially following instrumentation/procedures.

119. *Male: female is actually 10:1* and the disease is *uncommon* among caucasians. Early donovanosis may be mistaken for the primary chancre or condyloma latum of syphilis. In fact, in countries where donovanosis is endemic, the persistence of suspected condylomata lata after appropriate penicillin therapy for syphilis is highly suggestive of donovanosis.

123. In aminoglycoside toxicity, magnesium, K+, and calcium ***wasting*** is the rule.

126. This patient has ABPA (allergic bronchopulmonary aspergillosis). While indeed, aspergillus is a frequent colonizer of the respiratory tract, the presentation with wheezing, brown mucus plugs, high IgE and high blood eosinophils is highly consistent with ABPA. A common mistake is to start anti-fungals. There is no role for antifungal therapy in ABPA. Treatment is ***steroids***.

127. Itraconazole is the primary drug of choice for cutaneous/lymphonodular involvement in sporotrichosis. Lugal solution (saturated solution of potassium iodide) is the alternative treatment only.

128. Coccidioidomycosis meningitis is treated with fluconazole as the primary drug of choice.

129. In mucormycosis coma is due to ***direct invasion*** of the frontal lobe.

130. Acute toxoplasma infection evokes a cascade of protective immune responses in the normal host. Toxoplasma enters the host at the *gut mucosal level* and evokes the production of IgA antibody. Titers of serum IgA antibody directed at p30 (SAG-1) have been shown to be a useful marker of congenital and acute toxoplasmosis.

131. An important and common complication of severe malaria, hypoglycemia is associated with a poor prognosis and is particularly problematic in children and pregnant women. Hypoglycemia in malaria results from a failure of hepatic gluconeogenesis and an increase in the consumption of glucose by both host and parasite. To compound the situation, quinine and quinidine, the drugs of choice for the treatment of severe chloroquine-resistant malaria, are powerful stimulants of pancreatic insulin secretion. Hyperinsulinemic hypoglycemia is especially troublesome in pregnant women receiving quinine treatment. In severe disease, the clinical diagnosis of hypoglycemia is difficult as the usual physical signs (sweating, gooseflesh, tachycardia) are absent and the neurologic impairment caused by hypoglycemia cannot be distinguished from that caused by malaria.

137. Indeed, mefloquine is indicated for chloroquine-resistant areas *but is contraindicated in patients taking BETA-BLOCKERS.*

DERMATOLOGY

1-9. *Acanthosis nigricans* is not only associated with obesity ('pseudoacanthosis nigricans'), but is associated with a variety of insulin deficient states, such as diabetes, Cushing's disease, etc, and is also associated with various malignancies, such as gastric and ovarian.

Dermatomyositis also bears an association with gastric and ovarian carcinoma, as well as lung carcinoma. The malignancy may antedate or postdate the onset of the myositis by up to 2 years. The incidence of neoplasia is higher in patients over the age of 40 and is particularly high in patients over age 60; therefore, in such patients a thorough history and clinical examination (including breast, gynecologic, and rectal) should be supplemented by complete blood count, biochemical profile, serum protein electrophoresis and immunofixation, screening for carcinoembryonic antigen, urine analysis for blood and cytology, stool samples for occult blood, chest x-ray, sputum for cytology, and bone scan seeking clues for an underlying malignancy. This relatively inexpensive search uncovers most malignancies; undirected radiologic screening procedures are costly and unhelpful in improving the yield. The most common malignancies are lung, ovary, breast, gastrointestinal tract, and lymphoproliferative disorders.

In *erythema gyratum repens*, one sees hundreds of mobile concentric arcs and wavefronts that resemble the grain in wood. A search for an underlying malignancy is mandatory in a patient with this eruption.

Erythroderma is the term used when the majority of the skin surface is erythematous (red in color). There may be associated scale, erosions, or pustules as well as shedding of the hair and nails. Potential systemic manifestations include fever, chills, hypothermia, reactive lymphadenopathy, peripheral edema, hypoalbuminemia, and high-output cardiac failure. The major etiologies of erythroderma are (1) cutaneous diseases such as psoriasis and dermatitis, (2) drugs, (3) systemic diseases, most commonly Cutaneous T Cell Lymphoma (CTCL), and (4) idiopathic. The most common malignancy that is associated with erythroderma is CTCL. The patient may progress from isolated plaques and tumors, but more commonly the erythroderma is present throughout the course of the disease (Sezary syndrome). In the Sezary syndrome, there are circulating atypical T lymphocytes, pruritus, and lymphadenopathy. In cases of erythroderma where there is no apparent cause (idiopathic), longitudinal follow-up is mandatory to monitor for the possible development of CTCL. Other types of lymphoma can be associated with erythroderma, including Hodgkin's and non-Hodgkin's lymphoma, the former being more common.

The characteristic glucagonoma skin rash (*necrolytic migratory erythema*) is erythematous, raised, scaly, sometimes bullous, sometimes psoriatic, and ultimately crusted. It is located primarily on the face, abdomen, perineum, and distal extremities. After resolution, the regions of the acute eruption usually remain indurated and hyperpigmented.

Sweet's syndrome is characterized by red to red-brown plaques and nodules that are frequently painful and occur primarily on the head, neck, and upper extremities. The patients also have fever, neutrophilia, and a dense dermal infiltrate of neutrophils in the lesions. In approximately 10 percent of the patients there is an associated malignancy, most commonly AML. Sweet's syndrome also has been reported with lymphoma, chronic leukemia, myeloma, myelodysplastic syndromes, and solid tumors, primarily of the genitourinary tract.

10-18. The syndrome of *acrodermatitis enteropathica* includes severe desquamating skin lesions, intractable diarrhea, bizarre neurologic symptoms, variable combined immunodeficiency, and an often fatal outcome. This disease seems to be caused by an inborn error of metabolism resulting in malabsorption of dietary zinc and can be treated effectively by parenteral or large oral doses of zinc. Zinc deficiency might in part account for the immunodeficiency that accompanies severe malnutrition.

Dermatitis herpetiformis (DH) is an intensely pruritic, chronic papulovesicular skin disease characterized by lesions symmetrically distributed over extensor surfaces (i.e., elbows, knees, buttocks, back, scalp, and posterior neck). Because pruritus is prominent, patients may present with excoriations and crusted papules but no observable primary lesions. Almost all DH patients have an associated, usually subclinical, gluten-sensitive enteropathy.

Löfgren's syndrome, with which 5-10% of cases of acute sarcoidosis may present, includes E. nodosum, fever, arthralgias, and bilateral hilar lymphadenopathy.

Livedo reticularis is a mottled bluish (livid) discoloration of the skin that looks like a net. It is not a diagnosis per se, but more a reaction pattern to vasculitis syndromes, drugs, atheroemboli.

Lupus pernio is a particular type of sarcoidosis that involves the tip of the nose and the earlobes, with lesions that are violaceous in color rather than red-brown. This form of sarcoidosis is associated with involvement of the upper respiratory tract.

Morphea, which has been called localized scleroderma, is characterized by localized thickening and sclerosis of skin, usually affecting young adults or children. Morphea begins as erythematous or flesh-colored plaques that become sclerotic, develop central hypopigmentation, and demonstrate an erythematous border. In most cases, patients have one or a few lesions, and the disease is termed localized morphea. In some patients, widespread cutaneous lesions may occur, without systemic involvement. This form is called generalized morphea. Most patients with morphea do not have autoantibodies.

Necrobiosis lipoidica diabeticorum are the yellow-brown atrophic telangiectatic plaques that typically appear on the shins or other potential areas of trauma in diabetics.

35. Oral leukoplakia, which is associated with HPV-11 and HPV-16, is *not* the same thing as oral hairy leukoplakia, which is associated with EBV and is usually seen in advanced AIDS.

36. Basal cell ca, while malignant in its locally aggressive growth properties, bears a limited capacity to metastasize.

51. In HANE, there is no urticaria and the lesions are not pruritic. Not only does the swelling *not* respond to epinephrine, but it is a helpful means to differentiate common angioedema, which responds within minutes to epinephrine, and in which there is pruritis and urticaria.

74. Henoch-Schönlein purpura is a subtype of acute leukocytoclastic vasculitis that is seen primarily in children and adolescents following an upper respiratory infection. The majority of lesions are found on the lower extremities and buttocks. Systemic manifestations include fever, arthralgias (primarily of the knees and ankles), abdominal pain, gastrointestinal bleeding, and nephritis. Direct immunofluorescence examination shows deposits of IgA within dermal blood vessel walls. While palpable purpura are typically seen on the lower extremities and buttocks, there is no association with erythema nodosum.
75. The 5 types of Acanthosis Nigricans are:

    47 Hereditary benign AN: no associated endocrine disorder
    48 Benign AN: may be associated with insulin-resistant states (DM, acromegaly, Cushing's, Addison's and hypothyroidism)
    49 Pseudo-AN: complication of obesity (which is also associated with insulin resistance)
    50 Drug-induced AN: OCPs, nicotinic acid (high dose)
    51 Malignant AN: adenoca (2/3 gastric)

76. Cutaneous T-cell Lymphoma (mycosis fungoides) is a *malignancy of helper T cells* (CD4+).

77. *Erythroderma* implies generalized redness of the skin, scaling and thickening of the skin (erythroderma). A "velvety, hyperpigmented rash" would better describe *acanthosis nigricans*.

78. High levels of cortisol increase susceptibility (e.g. Cushing's or exogenous steroids). Treatment includes antifungals, e.g. selenium sulfide or topical/systemic azoles (keto/itraconazole).

79. While medications (penicillin, sulfa, thiazides, and allopurinol) can indeed cause HV, isotretinoin and chlorpropamide are not among those.

80. Many students get these associations confused because they appear to overlap in aplastic anemia, since aplastic anemia can be triggered by PNH, parvovirus B-19, and Hep B and C. And of course, hairy cell leukemia typically presents with cytopenias.

92. Unlike common acquired nevi, new lesions *continue to develop* over many years and after middle age.

93. This rash of NME indeed involves the central 1/3rd face, groin, perineum & lower abdomen but involves FLEXURAL (not extensor) surfaces and frictional areas with blistering, hyperpigmentation.

94. In addition to the classic periorbital heliotrope rash and Gottren's papules overlying the knuckles, patients with dermatomyositis typically show photosensitivity and *poikiloderma*, a term used to describe a patch of skin with (1) reticulated hypo- and hyperpigmentation, (2) wrinkling secondary to epidermal atrophy, and (3) telangiectasias. Other dermatologic manifestations of dermatomyositis include:
    - Cuticular hypertrophy with punctate infarcts
    - Periungal telangiectasias
    - Calcinosis
    - Extensor erythema
    - In adults, the risk of ca is 5-7x increased. Associated malignancies include: *breast, ovary, uterus, lung, colon, stomach. Treatment of DM is steroids $\pm$ azathioprine.*

95. Primary **amyloidosis** and **amyloidosis** associated with multiple myeloma may involve the skin of the extremities and face diffusely to give the appearance of **scleroderma**. Biopsy will clearly differentiate these entities.

96. Icthyosis vulgaris is associated with atopic conditions, including atopic dermatitis, allergic rhinitis, and ***intrinsic*** asthma. In addition I.V. may also be seen in Non-Hodgkin's lymphoma, myeloma, Kaposi's sarcoma, and may be secondary to nicotinic acid.

97. **Associated with AML and febrile LOWER respiratory infections.** *Sweet's syndrome*, or *acute febrile neutrophilic dermatosis*, was originally described in women with elevated white blood cell counts. The disease is characterized by the presence of leukocytes in the lower dermis, with edema of the papillary body. Ironically, this disease now is usually seen in patients with neutropenic cancer, most often in association with acute leukemia but also in association with a variety of other malignancies. The edema may suggest vesicles, but on palpation the lesions are solid, and vesicles probably never arise in this disease. The lesions are most common on the face, neck, and arms. On the legs, they may be confused with erythema nodosum. The development of lesions is often accompanied by high fevers and an elevated erythrocyte sedimentation rate. Both the lesions and the temperature elevation respond dramatically to steroids.

98. *Nikolsky sign* describes when application of pressure to a preexisting blister causes extension of the bullae. Manual pressure to the skin of these patients may elicit the separation of the epidermis. This finding, while characteristic of PV, is not specific to this disorder and is also seen in toxic epidermal necrolysis, Stevens-Johnson syndrome, and a few other skin diseases.

99. Unlike pemphigus vulgaris, BP bears no association to malignancy.

100. Lupus pernio bears no association with either systemic or discoid lupus. It is simply the cutaneous manifestation of sarcoidosis.

101. Angioid streaks are found in the retina and represent rupture of Bruch's membrane secondary to an elastic fiber defect. These streaks are typically yellowish in color, wider than blood vessels, and extend across the fundus.

102. Because the clinical and histologic features of this disease can be variable and resemble other subepidermal blistering disorders, the diagnosis can be confirmed by direct *immunofluorescence* microscopy of normal-appearing perilesional skin. Such studies demonstrate granular deposits of IgA (with or without complement components) in the papillary dermis and along the epidermal basement membrane zone. IgA deposits in the skin are unaffected by control of disease with medication; however, these immunoreactants may diminish in intensity or disappear in patients maintained for long periods on a strict gluten-free diet (see below). Patients with granular deposits of IgA in their epidermal basement membrane zone typically do not have circulating IgA anti-basement membrane autoantibodies and should be distinguished from individuals with linear IgA deposits at this site. Despite the fact that Linear IgA Disease is also a bullous disease that is pruritic and involves IgA, it is not considered a variant of dermatitis herpetiformis.

103. Hereditary Hemorrhagic Telangiectasia, aka Osler-Weber-Rendu syndrome, is an autosomal dominant disease affecting blood vessels exclusively and does not involve abnormal platelet numbers of function. AVMs in the GI and pulmonary systems account for the majority of symptoms, including epistaxis, GI bleeds, and hemoptysis.

104. This disease can be treated effectively by parenteral *or large oral doses* of zinc.

105. The patient has Lyme disease. The rash is erythema chronicum migrans. He presents with the usual prodrome of symptoms that may also include arthralgias. Remember, ordering Lyme titres is not appropriate at this stage, since they usually won't be positive this early, and the diagnosis at this stage should be made based on the history and the characteristic rash. 14% of patients report a history of a tick bite. Removal of the tick <u>within 18 hours</u> may preclude infection.

106. Scleroderma, indeed, is usually classified into *limited* disease or *diffuse* disease.

Characteristics of each include:

- *Limited* (60%):
  - Usually female
  - Long h/o Raynaud's phenomenon usually
  - Acrosclerosis
  - CREST syndrome as well as Morphea falls here
  - Systemic involvement may not appear for years
  - High incidence of anticentromere Ab

- *Diffuse* (40%)
  - Relatively rapid onset; indeed diffuse
  - Anticentromere Ab uncommon, but Scl-70 in 30%
  - Internal organ involvement may be seen (heart, lungs, GI tract)

107. The female to male ratio is 3:1, not vice versa. Indeed there is some evidence that Borrelia burgdorferi may actually be the causative agent, at least in some patients. For morphea lesions not associated with borrelia burgdorferi, there is no effective tx beyond symptomatic as necessary; otherwise, high-dose parenteral PCN or Ceftriaxone regimens may reverse.

108. GVHD is an immune disorder caused by immunocompetent donor cells reacting vs. the tissues of an immunocompetent host. Chronic manifestations appear **> 100 days post transplant** and may arise either from acute disease or *de novo*. Acute manifestations include: fever, jaundice, serositis, pulmonary insufficiency, TEN, diarrhea, liver dysfunction. Treatment includes steroids; cyclosporine; PUVA.

109. Koplik's spots are indeed pathognomonic but are actually a cluster of *tiny bluish-white* papules appearing on or after 2nd day of febrile illness *on buccal mucosa opposite premolar teeth*. Spread of disease in *rubella*, on the other hand, is typically from face to trunk in about 1 day.

110. The patient has Rocky Mountain Spotted Fever. Areas endemic for this disease include Canada, Mexico, Costa Rica, Panama, Columbia, and Brazil. Typically the rash begins on the wrists, ankles, arms and spreads to the trunk ("centripetally", unlike measles), palms, and soles. It is caused by a tick bite (**W**ood tick=Dermacentor andersoni in the **W**estern US. Dog tick=D. variabilis in East) usually in mid-to-late summer. R. Rickettsii, of course, is the bacteria responsible for the disease. In the United States, the disease is relatively rare in Rocky Mountain states and is most common in mid-Atlantic states. Only 60% give a h/o a tick bite. Only 3% of cases with RMSF present with the triad of rash, fever, and a h/o a tick bite. On the *first* day of illness, only 14% of patients have the rash; during *first three* days only 49% have the rash; 20% take 6 or more days to see the rash; 13% have no rash (true "spotless RMSF").

As the disease progresses, patients may present with diffuse vasculitis, ***hyponatremia, thrombocytopenia***. Extensive cutaneous necrosis due to DIC occurs in 4%; these may become gangrenous. Diagnosis is via complement fixation titre or Weil-Felix DFA of a skin bx (false + in 30%); diagnosis should be made clinically and confirmed later (e.g. antibody titres). Treatment is with Doxycycline or TCN; chloramphenicol is an alternative.

111. Ecthyma gangrenosum, which usually starts as a cutaneous infection, progressing to infarction, bulla and finally to large ulcerated gangrenous lesion, is, in fact, usually solitary, but may be multiple. Seen in the setting of prolonged neutropenia, it is not uncommon to see pseudomonas aeruginosa bacteremia accompanying this necrotizing cellulitis.

112. Erisipelas is the *most common cause* of virulent soft tissue infection in a healthy host.

113. Erisipeloid is an acute but *slowly* evolving violaceous erythematous cellulitis usually to the hand 2° to Erysipelothrix rhusiopathiae after handling saltwater fish, shellfish, meat, hides, poultry. The rash is exactly as described, but enlarges peripherally with central fading. The term "erysipeloid" meaning "erysipelas-like" is due to the painful, swollen lesion with sharply defined irregular raised border.

114. The rash appears within 1-3 days of infection and erythema is first noted on the trunk and spreads to the extremities. *Palms and soles are usually spared of the rash despite the fact that exfoliation of the palms and soles usually follows the rash.*

115. Cat Scratch disease is a ***benign, self-limiting*** zoonotic infection that follows cat scratches or contact with a cat, and subsequent acute to subacute tender regional LN. Because it is self-limiting in most cases, ***antibiotics are usually not necessary***, and when they are, azithromycin can be used outpatient. Occasionally, surgical drainage of involved lymph nodes is required.

116. The patient has rosacea. Formerly, this was known as "acne rosacea" because of its acneiform appearance, even though it is actually unrelated to acne (though frequently coexists). Rosacea is a chronic acneiform disorder of the facial pilosebaceous units coupled with an increased reactivity of capillaries to heat, leading to flushing and ultimately to telangiectasias. Those at greatest risk include individuals of **Celtic or southern Italian descent.** Treatment involves either topical metronidazole or other topical antibiotics; if these fail or for more severe disease, PO TCN or minocycline may be used; if still those fail, then PO isotretinoin is an option. Avoidance of the patient's specific precipitating factors such as alcohol, hot or spicy foods, or significant stress, is also important.

117. This patient has Behçet's disease. The *pathergy test* is performed as follows: physician-placed oblique insertion of a 20-gauge needle under sterile conditions produces an inflammatory pustule at 24-48 h). It has nothing to do with the "anergy panel" or testing vs. fungal antigens. Remember, ocular disease occurs in 80% of patients with Behçet's , particularly in HLA-B5 patients and Japanese men. 98% have oral ulcers. 30% have thrombophlebitis. 30% develop colitis that is also more common in HLA-B5. When spondylitis/sacroiliitis are present in Behçet's, the patients are usually HLA-B27 positive.

118. While pulmonary KS can cause bronchospasm, intractable cough, progressive respiratory failure, SOB, GI involvement in KS *rarely* causes symptoms. At time of diagnosis, 40% of KS cases have GI involvement; 80% at autopsy. Pulmonary KS has a high mortality (median survival < 6 months). KS of the bowel/lungs is the cause of death in 10%-20% of AIDS patients.

119. The diagnosis is oral leukoplakia. Indeed, about 10% of lesions can progress to malignancy. However, lesions on the ***floor*** of the mouth are serious , with over 60% showing either carcinoma in situ or invasive SCC, *whereas* ***buccal*** involvement is almost always benign.

120. A multisystem disease with cutaneous lesions resembling urticaria, except that they *persist > 24 h, generally up to 3-4 days.*

121. The transverse white striae of the fingernails following arsenic poisoning are *Mee's lines.*

122. *While cutaneous photosensitivity is the major clinical feature in porphyria cutanea tarda (PCT), patients usually do not present with it.* Rather, patient usually present with complaints of "fragile skin", vesicles, and bullae, particularly on the dorsum of the hands, esp after minor trauma The porphyrias are inherited or acquired disorders of specific enzymes in the heme biosynthetic pathway. These disorders are classified as either hepatic or erythropoietic depending on the primary site of overproduction and accumulation of the porphyrin precursor or porphyrin, but some have overlapping features. The major manifestations of the hepatic porphyrias are neurologic, including abdominal pain, neuropathy, and mental disturbances, whereas the erythropoietic porphyrias characteristically cause cutaneous photosensitivity. The reason for neurologic involvement in the hepatic porphyrias is poorly understood. Cutaneous sensitivity to sunlight is due to the fact that excitation of excess porphyrins in the skin by long-wave ultraviolet light leads to cell damage, scarring, and deformation. Steroid hormones, drugs, and nutrition influence the production of porphyrin precursors and porphyrins, thereby precipitating or increasing the severity of some porphyrias.

123. Indeed, when differentiating variegate porphyria from PCT, besides the lack of acute symptoms, it is important to check the *stool for protoporphyrins* (neg in PCT, + in VP)

124. Essentially, pseudoporphyria is a vesiculobullous cutaneous condition that clinically and histologically resembles several of the features of PCT but is *devoid of biochemical porphyrin abnormalities.*

125. *Essential mixed cryoglobulinemia* (EMC), was reported initially to be associated with hepatitis B. The disorder is characterized clinically by arthritis and cutaneous vasculitis (palpable purpura) and serologically by the presence of circulating cryoprecipitable immune complexes of more than one immunoglobulin class. Many patients with this syndrome have chronic liver disease, but the association with HBV infection has always been controversial. Recent reevaluation of patients with EMC suggests instead that a substantial proportion have chronic HCV infection. Their circulating immune complexes contain HCV RNA at a concentration that exceeds its serum concentration; this observation argues against secondary trapping of HCV in the immune complexes and favors a primary role for the virus in the pathogenesis of EMC.

NEUROLOGY & GERIATRICS

1. The hearing loss in Meniere's disease is progressive and *sensorineural.*

2. About 15% of cases of myasthenia are associated with thymoma, and about 10% of patients with thymoma develop myasthenia.

3. GBS manifests as a severe, rapidly progressive, symmetric polyneuropathy indeed, but it starts distally and *ascends* with pronounced proximal muscle weakness. It is often described, therefore, as an ascending paralysis. Areflexia and a high spinal fluid protein level is also frequently seen.

4. Answer d) gives the common presentation for a herniated disk, which is certainly not an indication for *emergent* MRI.

5. Answer a) is describing, instead, *diabetic amyotrophy.*

8. *Cardioembolic sources of ischemic CVA include:*

MAJOR RISK FACTORS	MINOR RISK FACTORS
A Fib	MVP
Mitral Stenosis	Severe mitral annular calcification
Prosthetic valve	Patent foramen ovale
Recent MI	Atrial septal aneurysm
LV thrombus	Calcific AS
Atrial myxoma	LV regional wall abnormalities
Infectious endocarditis	
Nonischemic dilated cardiomyopathy	
Nonbacterial thrombotic endocarditis	
Sick sinus syndrome	

9. The commonest cause of spontaneous SAH is a ruptured saccular aneurysm. Aneurysms can undergo small ruptures and leaks of blood into the subarachnoid space, so-called warning leaks. Sudden unexplained headache at any location should raise suspicion of SAH and be investigated because a major hemorrhage may be imminent. <u>Most</u> aneurysms, however, present <u>without warning</u> as <u>sudden</u> SAH. Occasionally, prodromal symptoms suggest the location of a progressively enlarging unruptured aneurysm. A *third cranial nerve palsy*, particularly when associated with pupillary dilatation, loss of light reflex, and focal pain above or behind the eye, may occur with an expanding aneurysm at the junction of the posterior communicating artery and the internal carotid artery. A *sixth nerve palsy* may indicate an aneurysm in the cavernous sinus, and visual field defects can occur with an expanding supraclinoid carotid aneurysm.

Occipital and posterior cervical pain may signal a posterior inferior cerebellar artery (PICA) or anterior inferior cerebellar artery (AICA) aneurysm. Pain in or behind the eye and in the low temple can occur with an expanding middle cerebral aneurysm. Head pains in the absence of neurologic symptoms and signs are rarely caused by growing aneurysms.

19. Included among the differentials of facial nerve palsy is *Ramsay-Hunt syndrome*. The Ramsay Hunt syndrome, presumably due to herpes ***zoster*** of the geniculate ganglion, consists of a severe facial palsy associated with a vesicular eruption in the pharynx, external auditory canal, and other parts of the cranial integument; often the eighth cranial nerve is affected as well.

20-25. The most striking disorder of trigeminal nerve function is *trigeminal neuralgia*, or tic douloureux, a condition characterized by excruciating paroxysms of pain in the lips, gums, cheek, or chin and, very rarely, in the distribution of the ophthalmic division of the fifth nerve. The disorder occurs almost exclusively in middle-aged and elderly persons. The pain seldom lasts more than a few seconds or a minute or two but may be so intense that the patient winces, hence the term *tic.*

The most debilitating complication of herpes zoster, in both the normal and the immunocompromised host, is pain associated with acute neuritis and *postherpetic neuralgia*. Postherpetic neuralgia is uncommon in young individuals; however, at least 50 percent of patients over age 50 with zoster report some degree of pain in the involved dermatome months after the resolution of cutaneous disease. Changes in sensation in the dermatome, resulting in either hypo- or hyperesthesia, are common.

26-29. *Otosclerosis is a common example of conduction deafness. Acoustic neuroma is a classic example of nerve deafness.*

Essentially in the *Rinne test* holding the tuning fork against the mastoid process, the patient indicates when s/he can no longer hear the sound. At that point the tuning fork is changed to just outside the auditory meatus to see if the sound can be heard again. Normal hearing patients and patients with sensorineural hearing loss hear the sound longer through air than through bone, noted as "AC>BC" (air conduction > bone conduction). In a conductive hearing loss, bone conduction becomes ≥ air conduction, paradoxically. This result is reported as an "abnormal Rinne" or "reversed Rinne".

In the *Weber test* holding the tuning fork on the middle of the patient's forehead, the patient is asked, "Where do you hear the sound the loudest?" The sound localizes toward the side with conducting loss (toward the worse-hearing ear) or away from the side with a sensorineural loss (toward the better hearing ear). The Weber test is only useful if there is an asymmetric hearing loss. If hearing is symmetric, the patient perceives the sound in the middle of the forehead.

30. In determining brain death, if brain stem reflexes are present OR if they are persistently absent, there is no need to order an EEG.

35. Other conditions that predispose to cerebral aneurysms include essential hypertension, Wegener's granulomatosis, PAN, and SBE.

36. *A patient's failure to respond to one dopamine antagonist does not mean that s/he will not benefit from another.* Several dopamine antagonists are available. They are somewhat less effective than L-Dopa but are less prone to induce dyskinesias. Anticholinergics are the oldest group of PD medications and most effective in persons with tremor-predominant disease. Consider surgery for the patient only after medical therapies fail to confer benefit. Palliative surgeries, such as pallidotomy and thalamic deep brain stimulator implantation as well as so-called "restorative" surgeries, such as fetal mesencephalic cell transplantation are a few of the surgical options available to such individuals.

41. The patient has *progressive supranuclear palsy. Indeed, SNP may mimic Parkinson's disease (PD) in most ways.* Tremor, however, is unusual. The combination of supranuclear ophthalmoplegia and axial rigidity accounts for the common presenting complaint of frequent falls. The marked impairment of voluntary downward and horizontal gaze distinguishes this disorder from Parkinson's disease, as does the extended rather than flexed dystonic posturing of the axial musculature, the absence of tremor, and the poor response to antiparkinsonian medications. The course is generally progressive, with aspiration leading to a fatal outcome within 10 years. The response to pharmacotherapy is usually disappointing.

50. This patient has *multiple sclerosis*. Patients frequently note ↑exacerbations in hot weather. Symptoms associated with MS include: visual changes (including blurring, pain on movement, double vision); bowel/bladder/sexual dysfunction; cognitive deficits; depression and labile mood (mood swings); fatigue; impaired mobility; pain; sensory changes; spasticity; speech/swallowing trouble; tremor; visual changes; weakness. The most common initial symptoms are weakness in one or more limbs, visual blurring due to optic neuritis, sensory disturbances, diplopia, and ataxia. Cerebellar involvement results in ataxia of gait and limbs. In advanced MS, cerebellar dysarthria (scanning speech) is common. Sensory symptoms include paresthesia (tingling, "pins and needles," or painful burning) or hypesthesia (numbness or a "dead" feeling). Sensory symptoms often begin in a focal area of a limb, the torso, or the head and spread over hours or days to adjacent ipsilateral or contralateral areas of the body. Common optic findings include: 1) diplopia (usually 2° to INO, or internuclear opthalmoplegia); 2) optic neuritis (pain on ocular movement); and 3) nystagmus. Optic neuritis, common in MS, produces variable visual loss. It usually begins as blurring of the central visual field, which may remain mild or progress to severe visual loss, or, rarely, to complete loss of light perception. In mild cases, the patient may complain only of a subjective loss of brightness in the affected eye. Symptoms are generally monocular, but attacks may be bilateral. Pain, localized to the orbit or supraorbital area, is frequently present and may precede visual loss. The pain typically worsens with eye movement. Visual blurring in MS may result from optic neuritis or diplopia.

These two causes are distinguished by asking the patient to cover each eye sequentially and observing whether the visual difficulty clears. Diplopia in MS is often due to an internuclear ophthalmoplegia (INO) or to a sixth nerve palsy; ocular muscle palsies due to involvement of the third or fourth cranial nerve are rare. An INO consists of a delay or complete loss of adduction on attempted horizontal gaze to one side accompanied by nystagmus in the abducting eye.

56 & 58. The Argyll-Robertson pupil, seen in syphilis, is also known as the "prostitute's pupil", since it is said to "*accommodate* but doesn't *react*". Nevertheless, the pupil is still relatively small. When the near stimulus is removed, the pupil redilates very slowly compared with the normal pupil, hence the term *tonic pupil*. In Adie's syndrome, a tonic pupil occurs in conjunction with weak or absent tendon reflexes in the lower extremities. This benign disorder, which occurs predominantly in healthy young women, is assumed to represent a mild dysautonomia. Tonic pupils are also associated with Shy-Drager syndrome, segmental hypohidrosis, diabetes, and amyloidosis.

72. Patients with RLS improve with activity, like getting up and walking around. In contrast, paresthesia secondary to peripheral neuropathy persists with activity.

GERIATRICS

1-6. *The following is a useful summary of the features discussed in this question set:*

URINARY INCONTINENCE:			
TYPE	**PRESENTATION**	**ASSOCIATED FINDINGS**	**PATHOPHYSIOLOGY**
Stress	Small amounts of leaking with stress (***coughing, sneezing, laughing*, or *physical activity*** such as bending)	Multiparity; Estrogen deficiency Prior urethral procedure or radiation	***Urethral hypermobility; internal sphinctor deficiency***
Urge	***Sudden***, uncontrollable need to void resulting in loss of large amount of urine; ***nocturia*** and frequency also common	*Motor urgency:* CNS-related (CVA, Alzheimer's Dz, Parkinson's Dz, MS); spinal cord pathology; *Sensory urgency:* local bladder pathology or sudden ↑ in bladder volume (diuretic or glycosuria)	***Abnormal bladder contractions***; due to ***detrusor instability*** in a large % of these patients.
Overflow	Poor stream, straining, dribbling, although may present similar to urge or stress incontinence	***Obstruction*** (BPH, fecal impaction, tumor); ***Chronic bladder overdistension*** (such as from DM or detrusor areflexia)	**Bladder *overdistension***

7-8. *The effect of age on various labs can be seen in the following chart*:

↑ WITH AGE	↓ WITH AGE	NO EFFECT WITH AGE
Alk phos	Serum albumin	Bilirubin
Uric acid	Serum Mg	AST, ALT, GGTP
Total cholesterol	PaO_2	pH, $PaCO_2$
HDL	Creat clearance	serum creatinine
Triglycerides	T_3, TSH	T_4
Fasting blood glucose	WBC	Hgb, Hct, RBC indices, Plt
1h postprandial glucose	Vit B12	
2h postprandial glucose	CPK	
ESR		

9. Actually there is an *increase* in sleep latency with age. In addition to the correct features, there is an *advanced sleep-wake cycle*, that is, an earlier bedtime and earlier arising time.

10. Examples of *subcortical dementias* include Parkinson's disease; low-pressure hydrocephalus; MID (multi-infarct dementia). Subcortical dementias are characterized by prominent motor abnormalities and by changes in mood, personality, impulse control, and difficulty with planning. *Cortical dementias*, on the other hand, are characterized by disturbances in higher cortical functions that include language, calculation, visuospatial skills, and praxis (ability to follow commands). Alzheimer's is a good example.

ALLERGY & IMMUNOLOGY

2. The main cause of *anaphylactoid* reactions is radiocontrast media (75% of cases).
   Remember, anaphylact***oid*** reactions *resemble anaphylactic reactions in most ways, except they are not mediated by specific Ab (e.g. Ig E).* Because they are not mediated by IgE, skin tests are useless.

4. Despite common beliefs, there is no correlation between radiocontrast media reactions and shellfish or iodine allergies.

5-12. All of these relationships are summarized in the following table:

TYPE	MEDIATORS	EXAMPLES
I Immediate hypersensitivity (wheal-and-flare)	Specific IgE antibody	Allergic rhinitis Anaphylaxis; asthma urticaria
II Cytotoxic	Cytotoxic cells or specific Ab plus complement	Goodpasture's Graves' disease Myasthenia Gravis Immune hemolytic anemia and thrombocytopenia
III Immune complex (Arthrus reaction)	Specific IgG/M which complexes with circulating Ag and then complement	R.A.; SLE; Hep B viral prodrome
IV Delayed hypersensitivity (cell-mediated)	Specific T-cells that release lymphokines	Contact Dermatitis GVHD Response to TB/fungal/viral infections PPD testing

13. The opposite is true. RAST testing is *more specific, but less sensitive* than skin testing.

24-25. T cells are principally circulating and comprise most circulating normal lymphocytes. On the other hand, the majority of B cells are fixed and immobile, and only 20% circulate. T cells are generally *long-lived* memory cells, as opposed to the 2-3 day life-span of plasma cells.

CARDIOLOGY

2. Tall R-waves in V1 and V2 may be caused by:
    - i) Dextrocardia
    - ii) Hypertrophic cardiomyopathy
    - iii) Posterior wall MI
    - iv) RBBB
    - v) RVH
    - vi) WPW→ ✓ for delta wave
    - vii) RAD (right axis deviation)
    - viii) Rotation of heart (5% of population)
    - ix) Normal variant among young females

- ❖ Remember, left ***posterior*** fascicular block causes tall R-waves in the right precordium, since there is **right axis** deviation. Left ***anterior*** fascicular block is associated with **left axis** deviation.

4. Even though the 'c' in 'QTc' stands for 'calculated', you should really think of it as 'corrected' for the heart rate—because imagine the heart rate was at 300: the QT would be very short indeed! The QTc, therefore, takes the heart rate into account. So remember the rule of thumb to recognize ↑ QTc: If the QT interval (whatever the rate) is more than half the R-R interval, then the QT is prolonged.

This is a <u>very</u> important differential to remember for the exam:

- i) Ischemia: #1 cause
- ii) ↓Mg, ↓K+, ↓Ca; ↓thyroid
- iii) Pentamidine
- iv) Tricyclic antidepressants; phenothiazines
- v) IA Antiarrhythmics (e.g. PDQ: procainamide; disopyramide; quinidine)
- vi) Amiodarone
- vii) Any combination of Seldane with Erythro/Cisapride (pulled from the US market) /Azoles (e.g. ketoconazole)/Lovastatin

5. The chief coronary distributing blood to the posterior wall is the right coronary and the descending branch of the left circumflex artery.

6. The normal U wave is a small, rounded deflection (?1 mm) that follows the T wave and usually has the same polarity as the T wave. An abnormal increase in U-wave amplitude is most commonly due to drugs (e.g., quinidine, procainamide, disopyramide) or hypokalemia. Very prominent U waves are a marker of increased susceptibility to the *torsades de pointes* type of ventricular tachycardia . Inversion of the U wave in the precordial leads is abnormal and may be a subtle sign of ischemia.

7. In general, the height of the R-wave should ↑ as one moves across the precordium from V1→V6. Normally, you should see an R-wave height of 3mm by V3, or 4mm by V4. If not, that is called "poor R-wave progression" and is usually evidence of CAD. If V3R>V4R, on the other hand, that's called "*regression*", and that may be evidence of *infarct expansion*. Beware, however, that an EKG taken during a prolonged inspiration (heart moves away from chest wall leads) can simulate this, so should repeat on normal breathing. Large R's in the right precordium and deep S's in the left precordium would actually be what you'd expect to find in RVH. The criteria for *left* ventricular hypertrophy, by the way, are:

   i) R-wave in lead I ≥ 11mm
   ii) R-wave in aVL ≥ 12
   iii) S in V1/2 + R in V5/6 ≥ 35 (really any 2 precordial leads)
   iv) S in V2 ≥ 25
   v) R in I + S in III ≥ 25

9. **Absolute contraindications** include:
   1) Prior intracranial bleed or CNS tumor;
   2) Recent prolonged CPR;
   3) Active internal bleeding;
   4) *CVA or head trauma within the previous 6 months*;
   5) Use of streptokinase for the second time in a year (since patient builds up antibodies to it and tends to react poorly the second time if used so soon after.

   Relative contraindications include:
   1) GIB within 1 month;
   2) Surgery or trauma in the past 2 weeks;
   3) Pregnancy;
   4) BP >200/110.

11. ***Do not give* nitroprusside (Nipride) to patients wlth RVI**: it can markedly reduce the RV and therefore LV preload (primarily due to venodilatation) causing BP to drop dramatically. Efforts must be made to increase preload. RVI commonly accompanies posterior wall infarctions. The same goes for *Hypertrophic Cardiomyopathy,* by the way, in respect to volume dependence. Diuretics, nitrates, and other vasodilators should be avoided since in HCM they will *increase* the obstruction.

12. Remember to look for *T-wave inversions* ± ST *depressions* in unstable angina. ST elevations are not seen in unstable angina.

13. *Sino-atrial exit block and PAT with 2:1 block* are the two arrhythmias that reflect classic digoxin toxicity. The two arrhythmias that digoxin never causes are Mobitz II and atrial fibrillation.

14. Patients with *pacemaker syndrome* are, paradoxically, short of breath at rest, but relieved with exertion. Factors contributing to the pacemaker syndrome include (1) loss of atrial contribution to ventricular systole; (2) vasodepressor reflex initiated by cannon a waves, which are caused by atrial contractions against a closed tricuspid valve and observed in the jugular venous pulse; and (3) systemic and pulmonary venous regurgitation due to atrial contraction against a closed AV valve.

15. Remember, in LAFB, look for small Qs in I, L and deep S inferiorly. This is reversed in RAFB. Also, LEFT anterior fascicular block requires **L**AD> -45°, and RIGHT anterior fascicular block requires **R**AD> -45°.

16. From a management point of view, differentiating CHB and AVD is essentially semantics, since *both require a pacemaker.*

17. Cardiogenic shock can also occur after prolonged cardiopulmonary bypass; the ***stunned myocardium*** may require hours or days to recover sufficiently to support the circulation. Remember, stunned myocardium is usually seen in acute settings, like acute MI, and reflects the inability of the myocardium to make ATP (due to a problem in the Kreb's cycle). This is why an echo done too soon after an MI can give falsely low ejection fractions. ***Hibernating myocardium*** is a chronic problem reflecting hypoperfused myocardium with an intact Krebs cycle. It can be detected with thallium stress test, checking for "reversible defects", or using a PET scan (with agents such as F^{18}, $NH^{4}+$, etc.).

18. VSD, papillary muscle rupture, and refractory unstable angina are actually 3 of the key *indications* for using IABP.

19. Thyrotoxicosis, not hypothyroidism can cause ventricular bigeminy. Other important causes of ventricular bigeminy include hypoxia and electrolyte disturbances.

20. By definition, MAT requires three or more consecutive P waves of different morphologies at rates greater than 100 beats per minute. Remember, treatment of MAT includes verapamil, and of course, treating the underlying COPD. ***Patients should NOT receive digoxin unless MAT progresses to atrial fibrillation.*** There is a high incidence of atrial fibrillation (50 to 70 percent) in patients with MAT. Following theophylline administration, MAT is particularly common.

21. WAP has nothing to do with physically implanted pacemakers.

22. ASA decreases mortality/increases survival by 23% when used during an acute MI. Lytic therapy increases survival by approximately 20%; beta-blockers by 9%; and ACEI 3 days out by 7%. *Nitrates have only been shown to reduce morbidity, not mortality.*

23. You must know that ASD classically gives a fixed-split S2. This is in contrast to all the other types of split S2, which are listed below:

    i) Loud A2→systemic HTN
    ii) Narrow split with loud P2→Pulmonary HTN
    iii) Paradoxical (P2<A2)→LBBB
    iv) Physiologic—normally A2 is heard before P2, and this widens on inspiration.
    v) Single S2 (inaudible A2)→calcific AS
    vi) Wide split with soft P2→Pulmonary Stenosis
    vii) *Widely split*→RBBB

27-29.

	RA	PCWP	CO
RVI	↑↑	↓	↓↓
Tamponade	↑↑	↑↑	↓↓

One of the key ways to differentiate these two entities, therefore, is the wedge.

30. Know the clinical manifestations of tamponade: hypotension; JVD (and Kussmaul's sign)***; pulsus paradoxus***; ***electrical alternans***. In pulsus paradoxus, the decrease in systolic arterial pressure that normally accompanies the reduction in arterial pulse amplitude during inspiration is accentuated. In patients with pericardial tamponade, airway obstruction, or superior vena cava obstruction, the decrease in systolic arterial pressure frequently exceeds the normal decrease of 10 mmHg and the peripheral pulse may even disappear completely during inspiration.
    Entirely unrelated is ***pulsus alternans***, a pattern in which there is regular alteration of the pressure pulse amplitude, despite a regular rhythm. It is due to alternating left ventricular contractile force, usually denotes severe impairment of left ventricular function, and commonly occurs in patients who also have a loud third heart sound. Pulsus alternans also may occur during or following paroxysmal tachycardia or for several beats following a premature beat in patients without heart disease.

31. Know that *quinidine, verapamil, thiazides, erythro, & amiodarone* can ***increase the digoxin level***.

32. *Radiofrequency catheter ablation* of bypass tracts is the treatment of choice in patients with *symptomatic* arrhythmias. The diagnostic *triad* of ***WPW*** consists of a wide QRS complex associated with a relatively short PR interval and slurring of the initial part of the QRS (delta wave), the latter effect due to aberrant activation of ventricular myocardium. The presence of a bypass tract predisposes to reentrant supraventricular tachyarrhythmias. Know too that *procainamide* is the drug of choice for rate control when patients with WPW go into Afib or Aflutter.

Digitalis and intravenous verapamil are contraindicated in patients who have WPW syndrome plus AF, since these drugs can shorten the refractory period of the accessory pathway and can increase the ventricular rate, thereby placing the patient at increased risk for VF. EKG findings in WPW syndrome include: *short PR interval*; wide QRS complex; and slurring on the upstroke of the QRS produced by early ventricular activation over the bypass tract yielding the delta wave. Inferiorly, delta waves may appear as Q-waves, mimicking myocardial infarction—hence the term "*pseudoinfarction*" pattern.

34. Remember, there is a *decrease* in systemic vascular resistance in the third trimester of pregnancy. The changes in cardiac physiology during 3rd trimester therefore include an ↑ in blood *volume* and cardiac *output* (↑ stroke volume and heart rate); and a ↓ in *systemic vascular resistance*.

43-48. Anticoagulation In Nonvalvular AFib—Current Recommendations:

	Age <65	**Age 65-75**	**Age >75**
Risk factors for CVA	Warfarin	Warfarin	Warfarin
No risk factors	ASA	Warfarin or ASA	Warfarin

49-55. In contrast, a large, bounding (*hyperkinetic*) pulse is usually associated with an increased left ventricular stroke volume, a wide pulse pressure, and a decrease in peripheral vascular resistance. This pattern occurs characteristically in patients with an elevated stroke volume, as in complete heart block; with hyperkinetic circulation due to anxiety, anemia, exercise, or fever; or with a rapid runoff of blood from the arterial system (as caused by a patent ductus arteriosus or peripheral arteriovenous fistula). Patients with mitral regurgitation or a ventricular septal defect also may have a bounding pulse, since vigorous left ventricular ejection produces a rapid upstroke in the arterial pulse, even though the duration of systole and the forward stroke volume may be diminished. In aortic regurgitation, the rapidly rising, bounding arterial pulse results from an increased left ventricular stroke volume and an increased rate of ventricular ejection.

In aortic valve stenosis, the delayed systolic peak, *pulsus tardus*, results from obstruction to left ventricular ejection.

The *bisferiens pulse*, which has two systolic peaks, is characteristic of aortic regurgitation (with or without accompanying stenosis) and of hypertrophic cardiomyopathy. In the latter condition, the pulse wave upstroke rises rapidly and forcefully, producing the first systolic peak ("percussion wave"). A brief decline in pressure follows because of the sudden decrease in the rate of left ventricular ejection during midsystole, when severe obstruction often develops. This pressure trough is followed by a smaller and more slowly rising positive pulse wave ("tidal wave") produced by continued ventricular ejection and by reflected waves from the periphery.

The *dicrotic pulse* has two palpable waves, one in systole and one in diastole. It occurs most frequently in patients with a very low stroke volume, particularly in those with dilated cardiomyopathy.

Pulsus alternans is a pattern in which there is regular alteration of the pressure pulse amplitude, despite a regular rhythm. It is due to alternating left ventricular contractile force, usually denotes severe impairment of left ventricular function, and commonly occurs in patients who also have a loud third heart sound. Pulsus alternans also may occur during or following paroxysmal tachycardia or for several beats following a premature beat in patients without heart disease.

In *pulsus paradoxus*, the decrease in systolic arterial pressure that normally accompanies the reduction in arterial pulse amplitude during inspiration is accentuated. In patients with pericardial tamponade, airway obstruction, or superior vena cava obstruction, the decrease in systolic arterial pressure frequently exceeds the normal decrease of 10 mmHg and the peripheral pulse may disappear completely during inspiration

A small weak pulse, *pulsus parvus*, is common in conditions with a diminished left ventricular stroke volume, a narrow pulse pressure, and increased peripheral vascular resistance.

56-64. The normal JVP reflects phasic pressure changes in the right atrium and consists of two or sometimes three positive waves and two negative troughs. The positive presystolic *a* wave is produced by venous distention due to right atrial contraction and is the dominant wave in the JVP, particularly during inspiration. Large *a waves* indicate that the right atrium is contracting against an increased resistance, such as occurs with tricuspid stenosis or more commonly with increased resistance to right ventricular filling (pulmonary hypertension or pulmonic stenosis). Large *a* waves also occur during arrhythmias whenever the right atrium contracts while the tricuspid valve is closed by right ventricular systole. Such "cannon" *a* waves may occur regularly (as during junctional rhythm) or irregularly (as in atrioventricular dissociation with ventricular tachycardia or complete heart block). The *a* wave is absent in patients with atrial fibrillation, and there is an increased delay between the *a* wave and the carotid arterial pulse in patients with first-degree atrioventricular block.

The *c wave*, often observed in the JVP, is a positive wave produced by the bulging of the tricuspid valve into the right atrium during right ventricular isovolumetric systole and by the impact of the carotid artery adjacent to the jugular vein. The *x descent* is due both to atrial relaxation and to the downward displacement of the tricuspid valve during ventricular systole. The *x* descent wave during systole is often accentuated in patients with constrictive pericarditis , but this wave is reduced with right ventricular dilation and often is reversed in tricuspid regurgitation. The positive, late systolic *v wave* results from the increasing volume of blood in the right atrium during ventricular systole when the tricuspid valve is closed. Tricuspid regurgitation causes the *v* wave to be more prominent; when tricuspid regurgitation becomes severe, the combination of a prominent *v* wave and obliteration of the *x* descent results in a single large positive systolic wave. After the *v* wave peaks, the right atrial pressure falls because of the decreased bulging of the tricuspid valve into the right atrium as right ventricular pressure declines and the tricuspid valve opens.

This negative descending limb (the *y* descent of the JVP) is produced mainly by the opening of the tricuspid valve and the subsequent rapid inflow of blood into the right ventricle. A rapid, deep *y descent* in early diastole occurs with severe tricuspid regurgitation. A venous pulse characterized by a sharp *y* descent, a deep *y* trough, and a rapid ascent to the baseline is seen in patients with constrictive pericarditis or with severe right-sided heart failure and a high venous pressure. A slow *y* descent in the JVP suggests an obstruction to right ventricular filling, as occurs with tricuspid stenosis or right atrial myxoma.

Remember also *Kussmaul's sign* (an increase rather than the normal decrease in the CVP during inspiration) is most often caused by severe right-sided heart failure; it is a frequent finding in patients with constrictive pericarditis or right ventricular infarction.

65. Other conditions that can give a soft S1 include large pericardial effusion and mitral stenosis with a rigid valve. MS with a mobile valve, sinus tachycardia, and WPW all yield a loud S1.

74-75. Early systolic murmurs begin with S_1 and extend for a variable period of time, ending well before S_2. Their causes are relatively few in number. *Acute severe mitral regurgitation* into a normal-sized, relatively noncompliant left atrium results in an early and attenuated systolic murmur that is decrescendo in configuration and usually best heard at or just medial to the apical impulse. These characteristics reflect the rapid rise in left atrial pressure caused by the sudden volume load into a nondilated chamber and contrast sharply with the auscultatory features of chronic mitral regurgitation. Clinical settings in which this occurs include: (1) papillary muscle rupture complicating acute myocardial infarction, (2) infective endocarditis, (3) rupture of chordae tendinae, and (4) blunt chest wall trauma. MVP causes a late systolic murmur.

76. *Thrills* are palpable, low-frequency vibrations associated with heart murmurs. The systolic murmur of mitral regurgitation may be palpated at the cardiac apex. When the palm of the hand is placed over the precordium, the thrill of aortic stenosis crosses the palm toward the right side of the neck, while the thrill of pulmonic stenosis radiates more often to the left side of the neck. The thrill due to a ventricular septal defect is usually located in the third and fourth intercostal spaces near the left sternal border.

Acute mitral regurgitation from papillary muscle rupture usually accompanies an inferior, posterior, or lateral infarction. The murmur is associated with a precordial thrill in approximately one-half of cases and is to be distinguished from that associated with postinfarction ventricular septal rupture. The latter is more commonly (90 percent) accompanied by a thrill at the left sternal edge, is holosystolic, and complicates anterior infarctions as often as inferior-posterior events.

The recognition of either of these mechanical defects mandates aggressive medical stabilization and emergent surgical intervention

Ventricular septal defect produces a holosystolic murmur, the intensity of which varies inversely with the anatomic size of the defect. It is usually accompanied by a palpable thrill along the mid-left sternal border. The murmur of a ventricular septal defect is louder than that due to tricuspid regurgitation and does not share the latter's inspiratory increase in intensity or associated peripheral signs.

77. A loud S1 and the presence of an opening snap are indicative of valve mobility in MS. The *opening snap* (OS) is a brief, high-pitched, early diastolic sound which is usually due to stenosis of an AV valve, most often the mitral valve. It is generally heard best at the lower left sternal border and radiates well to the base of the heart. The A_2-OS interval is inversely related to the height of the mean left atrial pressure and ranges from 0.04 to 0.12 s. In the second intercostal space, an OS is often confused with P_2. However, careful auscultation will reveal both components of S_2, followed by the OS. The OS of tricuspid stenosis occurs later in diastole than the mitral OS and is often overlooked in patients with more prominent mitral valve disease.

78. When stenosis is marked, the diastolic murmur is *prolonged*, and the duration of the murmur is more reliable than its intensity as an index of the severity of valve obstruction. When a pulmonary insufficiency murmur and pulmonary HTN accompany severe MS, this is due to a *Graham Steell murmur.* This pulmonic valve regurgitation murmur begins with a loud (palpable) pulmonic closure sound (P_2) and is best heard in the pulmonic area with radiation along the left sternal border. Typically, it is high pitched, with a decrescendo quality, and is indicative of significant pulmonary artery hypertension with a diastolic pulmonary artery-right ventricular pressure gradient. Its increase in intensity with inspiration is a way to distinguish it from aortic regurgitation. The time interval between S_2 and the opening snap is inversely related to the left atrial-left ventricular pressure gradient.

The murmur is low pitched and best heard with the bell of the stethoscope over the apex, particularly in the left lateral decubitus position. While its intensity does not reflect the severity of the obstruction accurately, the <u>duration of the murmur</u> does provide some indication as to the magnitude of the obstruction.

79. Peripheral and coronary artery disease are the major cardiovascular associations of pseudoxanthoma elasticum. Ehlers-Danlos and Marfan's syndromes are, on the other hand, associated with MVP. Another connective tissue disorder, osteogenesis imperfecta (fragile bones, blue sclera) is associated only with aortic insufficiency. Other conditions associated with MVP include hypertrophic cardiomyopathy, ischemic or rheumatic heart disease, PAN, PCO, and WPW.

80-83. Remember, "*AS Failure*" to remind you that the order "Angina→ Syncope → (congestive heart) Failure" correlates to survivals of 3-5 years, 2 years, and ½-1 year respectively. Also, <u>*the later the peak*</u> of the systolic murmur→the worse the aortic stenosis. Similarly <u>*the loss of S2*</u> connotes a worse prognosis. Remember in AS, *valve areas* $\leq .75\ cm^2$ *are "critical"* stenoses.

84. Syncope of undetermined origin with clinically relevant, hemodynamically significant ***sustained VT or VF*** induced at EPS when drug therapy is ineffective, not tolerated, or not preferred. ICDs are *not* recommended for supraventricular arrhythmias.

85. Remember, however, that the *negative predictive value* of signal-average EKGs is much better than its positive predictive value, *so a normal SAE carries more weight as a good prognosticator than an abnormal SAE carries as a negative prognosticator.*

86. The ***adverse prognostic findings on exercise EKG* stress tests** are as follows:

- ↑ in complex ventricular ectopy (along with ST-segment shifts)
- Exercised-induced typical angina
- Low peak heart rate (e.g. <120 bpm without pacemaker)
- Low workload (e.g., <6.5 METs or 5-6min on Bruce protocol)
- Marked ST segment depression (eg. >2mm)
- Prolonged ST-segment depression (e.g. **>6min**) after exercise
- SBP ↓ (e.g. >10mm Hg from baseline) or flat response (peak<130mm Hg)
- ST-segment depression in multiple leads
- ST-segment elevation without abnormal Q wave

87. The following are characteristics of Cardiac Syndrome X:
- Exercise-induced chest pain, so + EST
- Atypical features of chest pain (e.g. prolonged episodes, poor response to sublingual nitrates)
- Negative stress echo
- Normal coronary angiogram
- Abnormal pain perception in many patients
- Microvascular angina in some patients
- Antianginals ineffective in ~ 50% of patients
- **Good** prognosis regarding survival
- More common in women with estrogen deficiency than those without deficiency.
- Still somewhat ill-defined

88. *Valvular hemolysis is a mechanical hemolysis and yields a negative Coomb's test.*

89. The statement *should* read: "Any patient with absolute *contraindication* to anticoagulation"!

90. *Digoxin ↑s the level of quinidine and verapamil by 50% and vice versa, so levels should be followed closely when used in conjunction. Verapamil and IV beta-blockers should not be used together secondary to an increased incidence of AV block.* Use of erythromycins in patients receiving chronic warfarin therapy may result in excessive prolongation of prothrombin time and increased risk of hemorrhage, especially in elderly patients, because of possible decreased warfarin metabolism and clearance; warfarin dosage adjustments may be necessary during and after therapy with erythromycins, and prothrombin times should be monitored closely. *An ACE inhibitor, like Vasotec, and a calcium channel blocker, like verapamil, are commonly used together and do not interact.*

91. While digoxin toxicity can lead to any bradycardia or block, it never causes Mobitz II.

92. Sick sinus syndrome is characterized by prolonged episodes of sinus *bradycardia* punctuated by paroxysmal bursts of Afib or flutter ('Tachy-brady' syndrome).

93. Caution should be employed when using digitalis or intravenous verapamil in patients with the WPW syndrome and AF, since these drugs can shorten the refractory period of the accessory pathway and can increase the ventricular rate, thereby placing the patient at increased risk for VF. In patients with the WPW syndrome and atrial fibrillation, DC cardioversion should be carried out if there is a life-threatening, rapid ventricular response. Alternatively, lidocaine (3 to 5 mg/kg) or ***procainamide*** (15 mg/kg) administered intravenously over 15 to 20 min will usually slow the ventricular response.

94. The benefits of digoxin are greatest in patients with severe CHF, an enlarged heart, and an S3.

95. PVD is a precaution only and certainly not a contraindication to the use of β-blockers.

99. Right heart cath is essentially another name for the "Swan" Ganz catheter commonly employed in the ICU/CCU settings, and has nothing to do with coronary catheterization which is, of course, done in a left heart catheterization study. The procedure is most commonly performed under fluoroscopic guidance using a balloon flotation catheter, which is advanced from a suitable vein (femoral, brachial, subclavian, or internal jugular) into the superior vena cava, where blood is sampled for oximetry. The catheter is then positioned in the right atrium, where pressure is measured. The balloon is inflated with air or carbon dioxide and advanced sequentially into the right ventricle, pulmonary artery, and pulmonary artery wedge positions. Pressures are recorded in each position. After the wedge pressure is recorded, the balloon is deflated so that pulmonary artery pressure can be monitored and blood samples can be obtained for oximetry.

With a thermistor-tipped balloon catheter, cardiac output can be measured using cold saline injection and a small computer (thermodilution technique). Comparison of oxygen saturations in the superior and inferior vena cava, chambers of the right heart, and pulmonary artery permits assessment of the presence of a left-to-right shunt at the atrial, ventricular, or pulmonary artery level, which will be manifested as an increase ("step-up") in oxygen saturation of blood as it traverses these vessels and chambers.

100. A *prominent x-descent* is seen in both cardiac tamponade (CT) and constrictive pericarditis (CP). On the other hand, a *prominent y-descent* is only present in CP. *Pericardial knock*, too, is only present in CP. *Kussmaul's sign* is another that is present in CP but not CT. On the other hand, *pulsus paradoxus* is absent in 2/3rd of CP, but is usually present in CT. In both conditions there is equalization of left and right ventricular diastolic pressures. However, in *constrictive pericarditis*, nearly all ventricular filling occurs shortly after mitral and tricuspid valve opening; after this period of rapid filling, ventricular volumes cannot increase further owing to the constricting pericardium. This abnormality produces an abrupt early ventricular diastolic pressure rise with a mid- and late-ventricular pressure plateau, giving the so-called *square root sign*. In contrast, in tamponade there is equalization of diastolic pressures with a gradual increase throughout diastole. Of note, *restrictive cardiomyopathy* can *also* give a square root sign.

106. In addition to those listed, patient monitoring with amiodarone includes chest auscultatory exam (recommended at periodic intervals; presence of rales, decreased breath sounds, or pleuritic friction rub may indicate pulmonary toxicity), bronchoscopy with lung biopsy, chest x-ray, EKG, ophthalmologic slit-lamp examinations, and amiodarone levels. BUN and creatinine are *not* a routine part of monitoring.

107. The murmur *increases* in hypertrophic cardiomyopathy with valsalva/standing/ nitrates (due to ↑ obstruction with ↓ venous return) and decreases with squatting/isometric exercises. Aortic stenosis shows the opposite.

108. EMD (Electrical-Mechanical Dissociation)—DDx: "HH PP TT" :

Cause		Usual Intervention
H hypertension	→	Bolus IVF
H ypoxia	→	Hyperventilate
P E	→	"
P H↓ (i.e. acidosis)	→	"
T ension pneumothorax	→	Chest tube
T amponade	→	Pericardiocentesis

115. *Carvedilol* is indicated, in conjunction with digitalis, diuretics, and/or angiotensin-converting enzyme (ACE) inhibitors, for the treatment of mild or moderate (New York Heart Association [NYHA] class II or III) heart failure of ischemic or cardiomyopathic origin, to slow the progression of disease as evidenced by cardiovascular *death*, cardiovascular hospitalization, or the need to adjust other heart failure medications.

116. Constipation is the most common side effect seen with verapamil. It is indicated, in conjunction with digitalis, diuretics, and/or angiotensin-converting enzyme (ACE) inhibitors, for the treatment of mild or moderate (New York Heart Association [NYHA] class II or III) heart failure of ischemic or cardiomyopathic origin, to slow the progression of disease as evidenced by cardiovascular death, cardiovascular hospitalization, or the need to adjust other heart failure medications.

117. Diagnosis may be had after a 3-day *high salt* diet, by measuring Na+, K+, creatinine, and aldosterone in a 24 h urine. a 24 h urine aldosterone >12 ng (if urine Na+>200meq) is diagnostic.

118. ACE I are *contraindicated in pregnancy*! In humans, ACE inhibitors can cause fetal and neonatal morbidity and mortality when administered in pregnancy. ACE inhibitors should be discontinued as soon as possible when pregnancy is detected. ACE inhibitors cross the placenta. Fetal exposure to ACE inhibitors during the second and third trimesters can cause hypotension, renal failure, anuria, skull hypoplasia, and even death in the newborn. Maternal oligohydramnios has also been reported, probably reflecting decreasing fetal renal function.

119. The use of nitroprusside may results in cyanotoxicity if thiocyanate levels are not checked every *48 hours*.

129-137. These findings, and others, are summarized in the table that follows ...

THE HYPERLIPIDEMIAS				
	PROBLEM	**PLASMA**	**PRESENTATIONS**	**TREATMENT**
Type I	Deficiency of lipoprotein lipase	↑ TG; ↑ chylomicrons; Creamy layer of supernatant after overnight incubation	➢ ***Eruptive*** xanthomas ➢ Pancreatitis	Fat free diet, medium chain TG, + fat-soluble vitamins
Type IIA	Deficiency of LDL receptors or overproduction of Apo B	↑LDL ↑TC	➢ ***Tendon*** xanthomas ➢ Premature atherosclerosis and CAD	HMG CoA reductase inhibitors + bile acid binding resins
Type IIB	↓ LDL and VLDL receptors	↑LDL ↑VLDL	Mixed	HMG CoA reductase inhibitors or nicotinic acid
Type III	Abnormal Apolipoprotein E	↑LDL ↑VLDL	➢ ***Palmar & tuberous*** xanthomas; ➢ Premature atherosclerosis and CAD; DM; hypothyroidism	HMG CoA reductase inhibitors or nicotinic acid
Type IV	Overproduction of Apo B and VLDL	↑ VLDL	Premature atherosclerosis and CAD	Gemfibrozil or nicotinic acid
Type V	Mixed I + IV	↑Chylomicrons; ↑VLDL; Creamy supernatant after overnight incubation	➢ ***Eruptive*** xanthomas ➢ Pancreatitis ➢ CAD	Gemfibrozil and/or nicotinic acid + low fat diet

PULMONARY MEDICINE & CRITICAL CARE

1-4. Remember for the exam (!) → ≥ **5mm** is used for 1) HIV+ patients; 2) recent contacts with active TB; 3) CXR shows evidence of prior but not active TB; and 4) Organ transplant recipients and similarly immunosuppressed patients on ≥15 mg prednisone for ≥ 1month. **At least 10mm** is needed for basically every other risk factor (healthcare workers, silicosis, diabetes, residents and employees of prisons/(other!) long-term facilities/hospitals/homeless shelters, s/p gastrectomy or jejunoileal bypass, etc (see Sanford Guide for complete list). **15mm or more** is reserved for everyone else, i.e. patients *without* risk factors or who are *not* recent immigrants (within the last 5 years) from countries with a high prevalence of TB.

5. In Lӧeffler's syndrome, one sees peripheral blood eosinophilia and transient pulmonary infiltrates; *there is no wheezing.*

6. Hemoptysis is usually the presenting feature in Goodpasture's syndrome.

7. Simple erythromycin estolate and TMP/SMX ds remain the drugs of choice in the treatment of bordetella pertussis.

8. Legionnaires's disease manifests clinically with: weakness, malaise, high fever, cough, and diarrhea, relative bradycardia, and bilateral patchy infiltrates. Labs may reveal: ↓Na, ↓ Phos, ↑ WBC, ↑ LFTs. Diagnosis: √ Ab with IFA (Indirect Fluorescent Ab) test; ≥ 1:256 or a 4-fold ↑ in titre. Treatment: erythromycin ± rifampin; fluoroquinolone; or azithromycin.

9. In massive hemoptysis, the cause of death is usually *asphyxiation*, not exsanguination.

10. The genus chlamydia contains three species that infect humans: chlamydia psittaci, chlamydia trachomatis, and *chlamydia pneumoniae (formerly the TWAR agent).* C. pneumoniae is a fastidious chlamydial species that appears to be a frequent cause of upper respiratory tract infection and pneumonia, primarily in children and young adults, and is a cause of recurrent respiratory infections in older adults. No animal reservoir has been identified for C. pneumoniae; it appears to be a human pathogen spread via the respiratory route through close personal contact.

13. CF pulmonary disease is associated with numerous complications. Pneumothorax is common (>10 percent of patients). The production of small amounts of blood in sputum is common in CF patients with advanced pulmonary disease and appears to be associated with lung infection. Massive hemoptysis is life-threatening and difficult to localize bronchoscopically. With advanced lung disease, digital clubbing becomes evident in virtually all patients with CF. As late events, respiratory failure and cor pulmonale are prominent features of CF. Patients with CF are not at higher risk for developing bronchopulmonary fistulas.

17. AP usually presents insidiously with dyspnea and cough. One third of patients are asymptomatic at time of diagnosis. The presentation is certainly not acute.

18. This patient has asbestosis. There is an increased incidence of ***adeno and squamous*** cell carcinoma. Radiologically, one can also see a pseudotumor presentation, called "round atelectasis" secondary to pleural thickening with an irregular zone of peripheral lung atelectasis immediately adjacent to it. It is caused when pleural effusion leads to an atelectatic segment (radiographically seen as "comet tail": due to blood vessels, bronchi coursing toward the mass).

19. Patients suspected of having mesothelioma must undergo an open pleural biopsy, as mesothelioma can "track" or "seed" along needle sites as well as chest tube insertion sites.

20. Remember, the treatment of ABPA is *not with antifungals.* Steroids, on the other hand, are critical in treatment.

21. Remember bronchorrhea (up to 8L/day !) is a characteristic feature for bronchioloalveolar carcinoma.

22. Most patients respond to steroids, often dramatically. BOOP generally has a favorable diagnosis.

34. In Caplan's syndrome, pulmonary nodules do indeed coincide with the appearance of nodules elsewhere.

35. Prognosis is usually excellent with conservative resection yielding an 87% 10-yr survival.

36. Unlike simple CWP, *PMF can progress* in the absence of further exposure, and in this way *resembles silicosis.*

37. Pleuritis/pleural effusion are more common than the rheumatoid pulmonary nodules. Nodules are usually associated with more severe disease.

38. Eosinophilic granuloma is most common in young caucasian males (M:F, 3:1) and is rare in blacks.

39. This patient has suffered a fat embolism and his presentation several days following his injury to the long bones is classic. Cerebral fat embolism causes cerebral purpura, mainly in the white matter, due to capillary occlusion by fat globules. There is evidence that patients in whom this complication is recognized and treated early have a better prognosis. Massive doses of glucocorticoids and administration of positive-pressure ventilation with high end-expiratory pressures have been claimed to be useful. Heparin or intravenous alcohol are no longer recommended.

40. Anti-GBM disease commonly presents with hematuria, nephritic urinary sediment, subnephrotic proteinuria, and rapidly progressive renal failure over weeks, with or without pulmonary hemorrhage. When pulmonary hemorrhage occurs, it usually predates nephritis by weeks or months. Hemoptysis can vary from fluffy pulmonary infiltrates on chest x-ray and mild dyspnea on exertion to life-threatening pulmonary hemorrhage. Hypertension is unusual and occurs in fewer than 20 percent of cases.

41. Detection of fat, usually by computerized tomography, is *pathognomonic* and *spares the patient from thoracotomy.*

42. Hypersensitivity pneumonitis, or extrinsic allergic alveolitis, is an immunologically induced inflammation of the lung parenchyma, involving alveolar walls and terminal airways, secondary to repeated inhalation of a variety of organic or other agents by a susceptible host. The diagnosis in most cases is established by (1) consistent history, physical findings, pulmonary function tests, and chest x-ray; (2) exposure to a recognized antigen; and (3) finding an antibody to that antigen. In a few circumstances, bronchoalveolar lavage and/or lung biopsy may be needed.

    Examination for *serum precipitins* against suspected is an important part of the diagnostic workup and should be performed on any patient with interstitial lung disease, especially if a suggestive exposure history is elicited. If found, precipitins indicate sufficient exposure to the causative agent for generation of an immunologic response. The diagnosis of HP is not established solely by the presence of precipitins, however, as precipitins are found in sera of many individuals exposed to appropriate antigens who demonstrate no other evidence of HP. Bronchoalveolar lavage in patients with HP consistently demonstrates an increase in T lymphocytes in lavage fluid (a finding that is also observed in patients with other granulomatous lung disorders). Following acute exposure to antigen, neutrophilia and lymphopenia are frequently present. Eosinophilia is not a feature. *Other examples of HP*, besides farmer's lung, include bird-fancier's (handlers) lung from exposure to pigeons, parakeets, and parrots; byssinosis in cotton handlers; and silo-filler's disease secondary to nitrogen dioxide.

43. It's the opposite. Cavitating mets are classically from squamous cell carcinoma, while >75% of lymphangitic mets are accounted for by adenocarcinoma. The adenocarcinomas are usually from lung primary, although other adenoca primaries include breast and GI. The mortality in lymphangitic spread is high (< 6 months). Lymphangitic mets often yield a normal CXR, but abnormal perfusion on V/Q.

44. Although pemphigus has been associated with several autoimmune diseases, its association with thymoma and/or myasthenia gravis is particularly notable (especially for the exam!) and this association is particularly true for pemphigus foliaceus.

45. Patients with Kartagener's do not suffer from pancreatic insufficiency.

46. Ventricular arrhythmias 2° to prolonged periods of apnea at night. Peripheral edema is 2° to pulmonary HTN/cor pulmonale. Anemia is not seen. In fact, polycythemia is seen 2° to $\downarrow pO_2$.

47. Hypoxemia is commonly ***exacerbated by*** exercise (similar to PCP).

48. Serum ACE levels may be elevated in many other conditions including hyperparathyroidism (which also causes hypercalcemia of course), mycoses (which can cause cough and E. nodosum), and a variety of other conditions. Non-caseating granulomas are certainly not specific for sarcoidosis and may be seen on other conditions that also cause hilar adenopathy.

49. Stage III, remember, is a bit paradoxical with pulmonary parenchymal disease without hilar adenopathy, i.e. there is "regression" of lymphadenopathy.

50. Additional indications for the use of steroids in sarcoidosis include ocular involvement, cardiac involvement, neurologic involvement, hypercalcemia, and disfiguring cutaneous manifestations (e.g. lupus pernio).

51. Amebiasis rarely manifests with pulmonary disease. Invasive amebiasis typically finds the liver. Furthermore, invasive amebiasis does not elicit eosinophilia.

52. Stonecutters and tunnel blasters are at increased risk for silicosis. When fever is present, one must suspect silicotuberculosis, and check a PPD. The disease can persist even after removing oneself from the source of silica exposure.

53. Mast cell stabilizers are considered second-line therapy in EIA, are effective in 70-85% of patients, but should be taken 10-45 min prior to exercise.

72. $FEF_{25\text{-}75}$ is the best measure of small airway disease when using PFTs. It signifies the volume of Forced Expiratory Flow that the patient exhales from ¼ of the way through his breath to ¾ of the way through his breath. In other words, it is the average expiratory flow rate during the middle 50 percent of the vital capacity and is also called the med-expiratory flow rate. The *$FEF_{25\text{-}75\%}$ is often considered a more sensitive measurement of early airflow obstruction, particularly in small airways.* However, this measurement must be interpreted cautiously in patients with abnormally small lungs (low TLC and VC). These patients exhale less air during forced expiration, and the $FEF_{25\text{-}75\%}$ may appear abnormal relative to the usual predicted value, even though it is normal relative to the size of the patient's lungs. With early obstructive disease, which originates in the small airways, FEV_1 /FVC may be normal; the only abnormalities noted on routine testing of pulmonary function may be a depression in $FEF_{25\text{-}75\%}$.

73. The main categories included in the differential diagnosis of an elevated A-a gradient can be remembered by the mnemonic "VSD", which is, in fact, one of the differentials: (see next) …

1. **V**/Q mismatching, e.g.
   a. PE
   b. Airway obstruction (asthma, COPD)
   c. Interstitial lung disease
   d. Alveolar disease
2. **S**hunt
   a. Intracardiac (e.g. **VSD!**)
   b. Intrapulmonary shunt (e.g. ARDS or intrapulmonary vascular shunt) and "intraalveolar filling" (pus=pneumonia; water=CHF; etc.)
   c. Alveolar collapse (atelectasis)
3. **D**iffusion defect, e.g.
   a. IPF
   b. Emphysema

As you can see, PE is *already* represented by the category V/Q mismatch and is not its own unique category.

74. Primary pulmonary HTN causes a ↓ DL_{CO}.

75. Goodpasture's syndrome causes an ↑ DL_{CO} . Diffusing capacity may be elevated if pulmonary blood volume is increased, as may be seen in congestive heart failure. However, once interstitial and alveolar edema ensue, the net DL_{CO} depends on the opposing influences of increased pulmonary capillary blood volume elevating DL_{CO} and pulmonary edema decreasing it. Finding an *elevated* DL_{CO} may be useful in the diagnosis of *alveolar hemorrhage*, as in Goodpasture's syndrome. Hemoglobin contained in erythrocytes in the alveolar lumen is capable of binding carbon monoxide, so the exhaled carbon monoxide concentration is diminished and the measured DL_{CO} is increased.

76. Empyema is exudative. Other exudative effusions include other pulmonary infections, pneumonia, pleural malignancy, and pulmonary embolus. PE can be *either* transudative or exudative.

78. There is no ↑ in pCO_2 with aging.

79. Several genes are associated with alterations in levels of serum α1AT, but the most common ones associated with emphysema are the Z and S genes. Individuals who are homozygous ZZ or SS have serum levels often near 0 but always less than 0.5 g/L and develop severe panacinar emphysema in the third and fourth decades of life. The panacinar process predominates at the lung ***bases***. The MZ and MS heterozygotes have intermediate levels of serum α1AT (i.e., between 0.5 and 2.5 g/L); hence the genetic expression is that of an autosomal codominant allele.

80. A D-dimer assay ***can help rule out*** PE in patients with nondiagnostic lung scans or a low pretest probability of disease:
    - For those patients with a low pretest probability of disease and a normal D-dimer result, the D-dimer assay has been shown to yield a *negative predictive value* of 99%.
    - For those with a nondiagnostic lung scan and a normal assay, the D-dimer assay has been shown to have a *negative predictive value* of 97%.

81. Pleuropulmonary manifestations, which are more commonly observed in men, include pleural disease, interstitial fibrosis, pleuropulmonary nodules, pneumonitis, and arteritis. Evidence of pleuritis is found commonly at autopsy, but symptomatic disease during life is infrequent. Typically, the pleural fluid contains very low levels of glucose in the absence of infection. Pleural fluid complement is also low compared with the serum level when these are related to the total protein concentration. Pulmonary fibrosis can produce impairment of the diffusing capacity of the lung. Pulmonary nodules may appear singly or in clusters. When they appear in individuals with pneumoconiosis, a diffuse nodular fibrotic process (*Caplan's syndrome*) may develop. Bronchiolitis obliterans +/- obstructing pneumonia may also be seen as a complication of rheumatoid arthritis. On occasion, pulmonary nodules may cavitate and produce a pneumothorax or bronchopleural fistula. Rarely, pulmonary hypertension secondary to obliteration of the pulmonary vasculature occurs. In addition to pleuropulmonary disease, upper airway obstruction from cricoarytenoid arthritis or laryngeal nodules may develop. There is no known association with spontaneous pulmonary hemorrhage.

82. Besides erythromycin and oral contraceptives, other medications that elevate the theophylline level include cimetidine, fluoroquinolones, digoxin, verapamil, propranolol, and allopurinol.

83. Remember, CEP shows diffuse interstitial infiltrates along the peripheral lung fields. When bilateral, therefore, this pattern is frequently referred to as the "photonegative" of pulmonary edema.

84. When the pO_2 is high, lower the FIO_2. Use the **Rule of 7's** to guide your adjustment in FIO_2: For every 1% decrease in FIO_2, the pO2 will drop by 7. So, for example, if the pO2 is 310 on 80% FIO_2, take 310-100 (goal)=210, which is the amount of decrease we will need to make in the pO_2. Dividing 210 by 7, we see we need to lower the FIO_2 by 30. So 80%-30% leaves **50%,** which is where we should order the new FIO_2 in order to bring down the pO_2 to 100. If the pO_2 is high and your FIO_2 is already low, then the PEEP can be lowered (usually in increments of 2 with follow-up blood gases). Because of oxygen toxicity, patients with a high pO_2 should have their FIO_2 lowered first, then the PEEP.

85. PEEP can cause a drop in the cardiac output by translating intraalveolar pressures to the pulmonary vasculature and ultimately limiting venous return to the right side of the heart, i.e. preload.

ENDOCRINOLOGY

1. Testicular feminization is the third most common cause of primary amenorrhea after gonadal dysgenesis and congenital absence of the vagina. The features are characteristic. Usually, a woman is ascertained either because of inguinal hernia (prepubertal) or primary amenorrhea (postpubertal). The development of the breasts, the habitus, and the distribution of body fat are female in character so that most have a truly feminine appearance. Axillary and pubic hair is absent or scanty, but some vulval hair is usually present. Scalp hair is that of a normal woman, and facial hair is absent. The external genitalia are unambiguously female, and the clitoris is normal. The vagina is short and blind-ending and may be absent or rudimentary. All internal genitalia are absent except for testes that contain normal Leydig cells and seminiferous tubules without spermatogenesis. The testes may be located in the abdomen, along the course of the inguinal canal, or in the labia majora. Patients tend to be rather tall, and bone age is normal. Psychosexual development is unmistakably female with regard to behavior, outlook, and maternal instincts.

2. Polycystic ovary syndrome (PCO) occurs in up to 20 percent of premenopausal women. In addition to the polycystic features of the ovaries, it is characterized by oligomenorrhea, hyperandrogenism, increased LH/FSH ratio, increased body mass index (BMI) within truncal-abdominal fat predominance, and an increased prevalence of insulin resistance.

3. In congenital adrenal hyperplasia (CAH), the LH/FSH is < 3:1, as opposed to PCO (Polycystic Ovary Syndrome, aka Stein-Leventhal syndrome) where the LH/FSH is usually > 3:1.

4. 21 hydroxylase deficiency is the most common form of CAH. The diagram on the next page displays the pathways of metabolism that reveal why patients *with 17α hydroxylase deficiency are frequently hypertensive and why 21 hydroxylase deficiency patients are frequently virilized*. The diagram thereafter illustrates the relationship between adrenal & gonadal sources of androgens, and the relationship between the cortisol and androgen synthesis pathways.

SYNTHESIS PATHWAYS OF CORTISOL AND TESTOSTERONE:

a thru c = enzymes, which you should *know for the exam*,

a = 17α-hydroxylase
b= 21-hydroxylase
c= 11β-hydroxylase

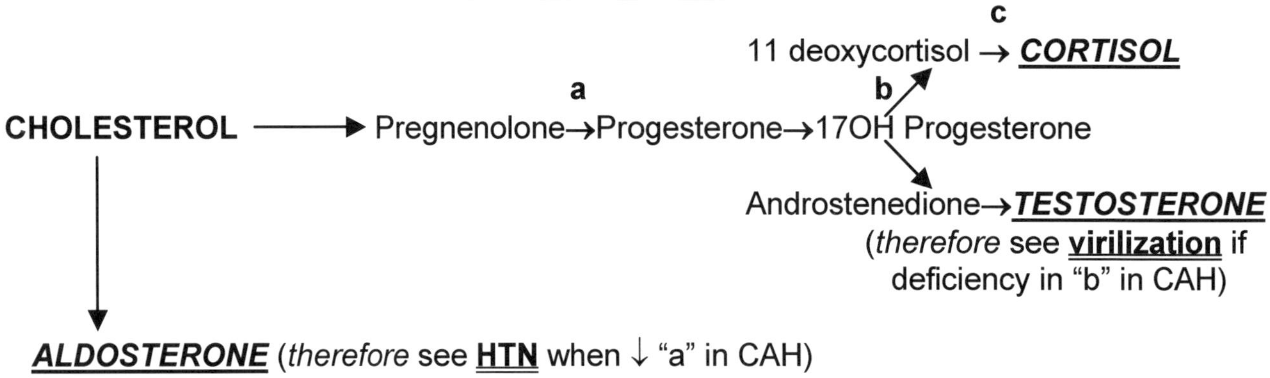

THE RELATIONSHIP BETWEEN THE CORTISOL AND ANDROGEN SYNTHESIS PATHWAYS: GONADAL & ADRENAL SOURCES OF ANDROGENS:

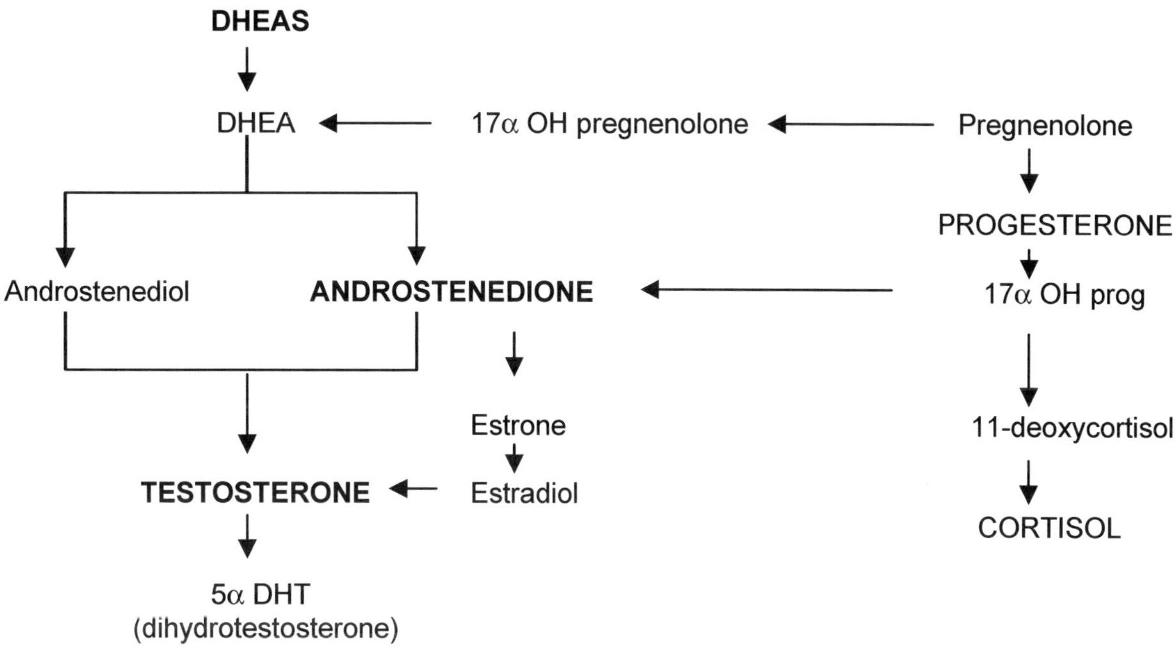

Therefore basic <u>initial</u> evaluation in hirsutism includes:

- **T**ESTOSTERONE
- **A**NDROSTENEDIONE
- **D**HEAS

...as in "she had a **TAD** too much hair."

6. The *clinical presentation* of acromegaly, a disorder of GH (IGF-1) excess, includes the following features:

    i) Acromegalic features
    ii) ***Carbohydrate intolerance*** in 20% ('PM SNAC' below will help you remember)
    iii) ↑ Sweating and oily Skin; skin tags
    iv) ↓ Heat tolerance
    v) Acroparesthesias
    vi) ***Carpal tunnel*** dz and other **N**erve entrapment syndromes
    vii) Prolactinemia (in up to half the cases), causing amenorrhea/↓libido/galactorrhea
    viii) ***Proximal myopathy***
    ix) Acanthosis nigricans (other causes of A.N. are obesity; DM; gastric ca)
    x) Sleep apnea
    xi) Cardiomyopathy or HTN

These might by remembered by using the following mnemonic: ***"PM SNAC"***: (**P**rolactinemia/**P**roximal **M**yalgia; **S**weating/oily **S**kin/**S**kin tags; **S**leep apnea; **N**europathies (entrapment); **A**cromegalic features/**A**croparesthesias; **A**canthosis Nigricans; **C**arbohydrate intolerance/**C**ardiomyopathy).

Diagnosis is made either by: 1) an ↑ serum IGF-1 (somatomedin); or 2) an OGTT (oral glucose tolerance test), checking for non-suppressible GH, i.e. GH that remains ↑ after administering ↑glucose load(this is the standard reference test). If GH does not suppress to < 10ug/L, the test is positive for GH excess. Mortality is ↑ 2° to HTN, DM, and cardiovascular effects.

7-13. Diabetes insipidus causes polyuria and polydipsia and may result from any of the following:

1. ↓Production of AVP→central DI→e.g. breast/lung ca mets, with ***abrupt*** onset of symptoms
2. ↓ Sensitivity of the kidneys to AVP→nephrogenic DI→e.g. ***Lithium*** toxicity
3. Functional suppression of AVP →primary polydipsia (compulsive water drinking)→e.g. a ***psych***iatric patient.

For proper diagnosis a ***water deprivation test*** is usually done ***first***. Essentially, the clinician deprives the patient of water and measures the subsequent urine and plasma osmolality. Normally, this would cause an individual to secrete ADH to conserve their water, causing elevations in subsequent measurements of serum and urine concentration. But in DI, there is either not enough ADH released from the brain or a lack of responsiveness to ADH at the level of the kidneys, so concentrations will not ↑ as expected to. Therefore, if the urine osm does not ↑ by >10%, the test is positive (for DI). ***Then***, the clinician can ***test with exogenous AVP*** to further clarify the source of the DI only if:

a) sequential urine osm vary by < 30 mosm /kg; or b) there is a 3-5% weight loss. Interpretation of the combination of these tests is summarized in the table that follows:

Water deprivation	Response to AVP	DIAGNOSIS
Normal	Absent	1° Polydipsia
+	**Present**	Central DI
+	**Absent**	Nephrogenic DI

Treatment depends on the cause…

a) Central DI→intranasal dDAVP (desmopressin)
b) Partial central DI→Chlorpropamide (AVP agonist)
c) Nephrogenic DI→Thiazides, but patient ***must be on a Na+ restricted diet*** to work

14-18. These findings could are summarized in the following diagram:

DIFFERENTIATING THYROIDITIS:

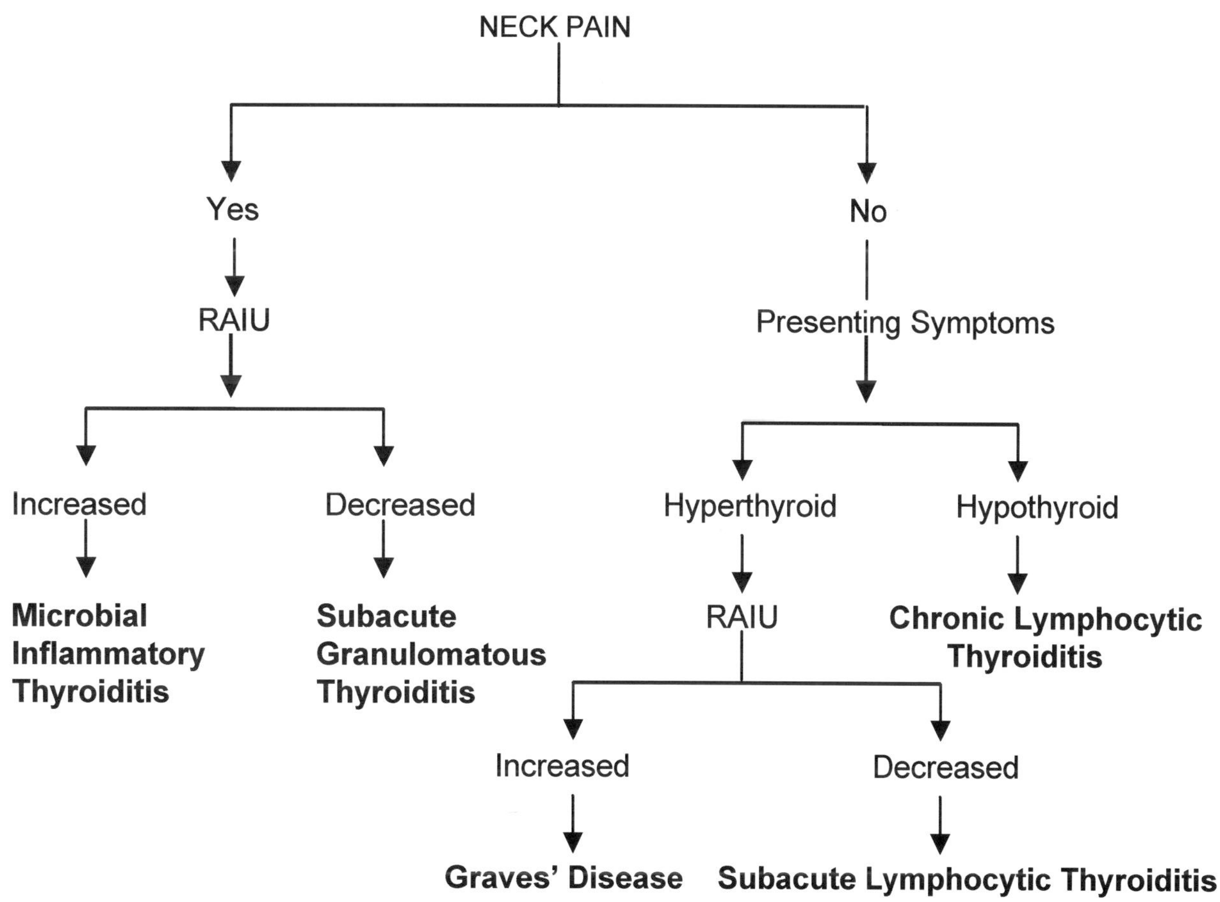

31. One valuable application of the RAIU test occurs *when thyrotoxicosis is associated with a low RAIU*. Causes include iodine-induced hyperthyroidism, thyrotoxicosis factitia, inadvertent ingestion of ground meat containing thyroid glands ("hamburger toxicosis"), and the spontaneously resolving thyrotoxicosis associated with painless chronic thyroiditis, postpartum thyroiditis, or subacute thyroiditis.

33. There is a general 90% rule of thumb for thyroid nodules:

    I. 90% are benign
    II. 90% (!) are "cold" (Note: only 20% of these are actually malignant; 1% for hot nodules)
    III. 90% are solid

    Indeed, hypofunctioning, hemorrhagic adenomas and thyroid cysts account for most of the cold nodules initially suspected of being carcinoma.

43. ↓T3 ↓T4 ↓sTSH (therefore it *can look like central hypothyroidism*, except may also see ↑*cortisol* levels in euthyroid sick) ; *free T4 is normal*; ↑ reverse T3.

44. TC is characterized by **hypo**tension.

45. Pretibial myxedema which manifests as waxy, infiltrated plaques is seen in patients with Graves' *thyrotoxicosis*, not hypothyroidism.

46. Osteomalacia is not seen. Remember, however, that hyperparathyroidism is a cause of secondary osteoporosis.

47. Urine calcium indeed is the key way to differentiate FHH and primary hyperparathyroidism. However, *urine calcium is low in FHH*, not high.

48. Thiazides cause a mild ↑serum Ca; and ↓ urine Ca (unlike other diuretics). Administration of thiazides can cause hypercalcemia in patients with high rates of bone turnover, such as patients with hypoparathyroidism treated with high doses of vitamin D. Traditionally, thiazides are associated with aggravation of hypercalcemia in primary hyperparathyroidism, but this effect can be seen in other high-bone-turnover states as well. Many aspects of thiazide action on calcium metabolism are unclear. Thiazides augment PTH responsiveness of bone and renal tubule. Chronic thiazide administration leads to reduction in urinary calcium; the hypocalciuric effect appears to reflect the enhancement of proximal tubular resorption of sodium and calcium in response to sodium depletion. Some of this renal action is due to augmentation of PTH action and is more pronounced in individuals with intact parathyroid secretion.
    However, thiazides cause hypocalciuria in hypoparathyroid patients on high-dose vitamin D and oral calcium replacement if sodium intake is restricted. This finding is the rationale for the use of thiazides as an adjunct to therapy in hypoparathyroid patients.

52. *Pseudopseudohypoparathyroidism is clinically very similar to pseudohypoparathyroidism, but without the biochemical markers*; i.e. part of the definition of pseudopseudohypoparathyroidism is in fact the absence of biochemical markers.

73. The most recent recommendations in the diagnosis of diabetes and abnormal glucose related states is summarized in the following table:

CRITERIA FOR DIAGNOSING DIABETES				
TEST	**RESULTS**			
	NORMAL	**IFG[1]**	**IGT[2]**	**DIABETES**
Fasting glucose	***<110***	110-125		***126***
Glucose intolerance (2h after 75g glucose load)	<***140***		140-199	200
Random glucose				200 with symptoms

[1] IFG, impaired fasting glucose
[2] IGT, impaired glucose intolerance

74. It is clinically important to make this relevant distinction, because the Somogyi phenomenon is avoided by ***decreasing*** insulin dosages for the critical time period, while the Dawn phenomenon usually requires ***increased*** insulin to maintain glucose in the normal range.

79. Remember, diabetic eye disease is divided into backround retinopathy (which includes hemorrhages, exudates, and microaneurysms), proliferative retinopathy (which includes the 3 correct answers here), and maculopathy. Remember, there is also an increased incidence of cataracts and glaucoma in diabetics.

80. Diabetic amyotrophy typically *spontaneously remits* after only 6-12 *months*.

81. Remember the inverse correlation between serum K^+ and pH. That's why bicarbonate is given with ↑ serum K+. In fact, bicarbonate should only be added if pH <7.2

The best way to monitor a patient with DKA for improvement is serial anion gaps, and not urine ketones which is less reliable due to the various types of ketones, not all of which are measured.

82-84. Cushing's ***disease***=2° disease at the level of the pituitary; caused by ACTH-producing tumor or hyperplasia. Cushing's ***syndrome***=1° disease at the level of the adrenal.

DIAGNOSIS:	**ACTH:**	**SUPPRESSIBLE WITH HIGH DOSE (8MG) DEXAMETHASONE?**
Disease (pituitary level)	↑	Y
Syndrome (adrenal level)	↓	N
Ectopic ACTH (e.g. tumors)	↑	N

Remember also, a 24 hour urine for free cortisol is the simplest screen for Cushing's syndrome. When testing using DST (Dexamethasone Suppression Test), the following are general guidelines:

- 1mg→is for **screening**; aka "**overnight** test" (or can do a 24h urine for free cortisol)
- 2mg→is for **confirmation**; the 2mg DST is aka "**low dose** DST"; a 2 day test.
- 8mg→is for **pinpointing** the exact cause; aka "**high dose** DST"; a 2 day test.

85. The presence of cortisol excess is suggested by the failure to suppress an 8 A.M. cortisol level to <140 nmol/L (<5 ug/dL) after an overnight dexamethasone suppression test (1 mg by mouth at midnight). Because there are many causes of false-positive failure of suppression, the diagnosis must be confirmed by the finding of increased excretion of urine free cortisol and/or 17-hydroxycorticosteroids that fails to decrease appropriately after 2-day low-dose dexamethasone administration (0.5 mg every 6 h for eight doses). Additional suppression (and occasionally stimulation) tests are required to determine whether the Cushing's syndrome is due to a pituitary lesion (Cushing's disease) or to some other cause. In patients with pituitary ACTH hypersecretion, high-dose overnight dexamethasone administration (8 mg at midnight) results in greater than 50 percent reduction in the 8 A.M. plasma cortisol level, and two-day dexamethasone administration (2 mg every 6 h for eight doses) should result in greater than 60 percent suppression of urine 17-hydroxycorticosteroids and more than 90 percent suppression of urine free cortisol.

86. Elevated vitamin D levels (>55) might point to sarcoidosis, ectopic production, and simple vit D intoxication. Normal levels at this point in the workup would point to endocrine disorders (such as hyperthyroidism, adrenal insufficiency, and pheochromocytoma), thiazides, milk-alkali syndrome, and increased bone turnover from immobilization, malignancy, hypervitaminosis A, and dialysis osteomalacia.

87-89. High C-peptide implies ***endogenous*** insulin secretion, which can result from either:

A. Insulinoma; or

B. Sulfonylurea abuse—this can be confirmed by simply checking sulfonylurea levels.

- Consequently, in hyperinsulinemic patients, the exclusion of sulfonylurea abuse points to insulinoma. Remember, sulfonylureas ↑ insulin secretion.

Low C-peptide, on the other hand, implies ***exogenous*** source, such as surreptitious insulin.

Elevated proinsulin reflects elevated endogenous insulin, as seen in insulinoma.

90. See the explanation to #4 in Endocrinology for the Synthesis Pathways of Cortisol And Testosterone.

NEPHROLOGY

10. In laxative abuse there is GI loss of bicarbonate which causes a metabolic acidosis, not alkalosis, and you only check *urine chloride in the workup of metabolic alkaloses*.

11. Hypokalemia secondary to renal potassium wasting, metabolic alkalosis, and normal to low blood pressure are the clinical features of Bartter's syndrome. Renin and aldosterone production are increased. Hypomagnesemia with hypermagnesuria may be present. Most cases are diagnosed during childhood, with the presenting symptoms, such as polyuria and weakness, being attributable to hypokalemia. Inheritance is autosomal recessive, though sporadic cases do occur. Although renal biopsy is rarely required for diagnosis, it reveals hyperplasia of the juxtaglomerular apparatus. Remember, in Bartter's syndrome, *because of pathology at the tubules, Na+ is lost, leading to volume loss, which in turn causes ↑renin →↑ aldo→↓K. The Blood Pressure is low/normal* despite the ↑ renin and ↑ aldo. It might help you to remember what's what if you already are comfortable with Type 4 RTA since they are practically ***opposites*** as seen below:

	Type 4 RTA	**Bartter's Syndrome**
Renin	↓	↑
Aldo	↓	↑
K+	↑	↓
BP	↑	↓/normal
Acid-base	Met. **acidosis** (non-AG)	Met. **Alkalosis** (Chloride-resistant)

12. Autosomal dominant polycystic kidney disease (ADPKD) has a prevalence of 1:300 to 1:1000 and accounts for approximately 10 percent of end-stage renal disease (ESRD) in the United States. Ninety percent of cases are inherited as an autosomal dominant trait, and approximately 10 percent are spontaneous mutations. The kidneys are grossly enlarged, with multiple cysts studding the surface of the kidney. The cysts contain straw-colored fluid that may become hemorrhagic. Only 1 to 5 percent of nephrons will develop cysts. The disease may present at any age but most frequently causes *symptoms* in the third or fourth decade. Patients may develop chronic flank pain from the mass effect of the enlarged kidneys. Acute pain indicates infection, urinary tract obstruction by clot or stone, or sudden hemorrhage into a cyst. Gross and microscopic hematuria are common, and impaired renal concentrating ability frequently leads to nocturia. Nephrolithiasis occurs in 15 to 20 percent of patients, calcium oxalate and uric acid stones being most common. Hypertension is found in 20 to 30 percent of children and up to 75 percent of adults. It is secondary to intrarenal ischemia from distortion of the renal architecture, leading to activation of the renin-angiotensin system. Urinary tract infections are common. Progressive decline in renal function is common, with approximately 50 percent of patients developing ESRD by age 60. However, there is considerable variation in age of

onset of renal failure, even within the same family. Hypertension, recurrent infections, male sex, and early age of diagnosis are related to early onset renal failure. Renal failure usually progresses slowly; if a sudden decrement in kidney function occurs, ureteral obstruction from stone, clot, or compression by a cyst are likely causes.

Patients usually have high hematocrits for their level of renal function, as erythropoietin production is high. Fluid overload is uncommon because of a tendency for renal salt wasting. *Extrarenal manifestations* of this disease are frequent and underscore the systemic nature of the defect. Hepatic cysts occur in 50 to 70 percent of patients. Cysts are generally asymptomatic, and liver function is normal, though women may develop massive hepatic cystic disease on occasion. Cyst formation has also been observed in the spleen, pancreas, and ovaries. Intracranial aneurysms are present in 5 to 10 percent of asymptomatic patients, with potential for permanent neurologic injury or death from subarachnoid hemorrhage. Screening of all ADPKD patients for aneurysms is not recommended, but patients with a family history of subarachnoid hemorrhage should be studied noninvasively with magnetic resonance imaging angiography. Colonic diverticular disease is the most common extrarenal abnormality, and patients are more likely to develop perforation than the general population with colonic diverticula. Mitral valve prolapse is found in 25 percent of patients, and the prevalence of aortic and tricuspid valve insufficiency is increased. Ultrasound is the preferred technique for diagnosis of symptomatic patients and for screening asymptomatic family members. At least three to five cysts in each kidney is the standard diagnostic criteria for ADPKD.

13. Hypocitraturia, not hypercitraturia, predisposes to calcium stone formation. Urine citrate prevents calcium stone formation by creating a soluble complex with calcium, effectively reducing free urine calcium. Hypocitraturia is found in 15 to 60 percent of stone formers, either as a single disorder or in combination with other metabolic abnormalities. It can be secondary to systemic disorders, such as RTA, chronic diarrheal illness, or hypokalemia, or it may be a primary disorder, in which case it is called idiopathic hypocitraturia. Treatment is with alkali, which increases urine citrate excretion; generally bicarbonate or citrate salts are used. Potassium salts are preferred as sodium loading increases urinary excretion of calcium, reducing the effectiveness of treatment. A recent randomized, placebo-controlled trial has demonstrated the effectiveness of potassium citrate in idiopathic hypocitraturia.

14. Measuring 24h urine for possible causes of nephrolithiasis is indicated in patients with recurrent stones, patients with a positive family history of renal stones, and patients who are either under 25 or over 60 years old.

86. Hypomagnesemia is associated with hypoparathyroidism, since Mg is needed for secretion of PTH by the parathyroid gland.

TOXICOLOGY

1. Isopropyl alcohol (rubbing alcohol) causes ketones and an osmolar gap but *NOT* an anion gap.

2. Remember, the half-life of opiates is a lot longer than the half-life of naloxone (Narcan®)! When naloxone is used to antagonize the effects of buprenorphine, butorphanol, nalbuphine, or pentazocine, larger doses may be needed than are required to antagonize the effects of most opioids having only agonist activity. When naloxone is used to treat opioid toxicity, continued monitoring of the patient is necessary after naloxone is administered. If the duration of action of the opioid exceeds that of naloxone, re-emergence of opioid toxicity following initial reversal is likely. *The naloxone challenge test* (recommended prior to initiation of naltrexone therapy in detoxified opioid addicts) should *not* be administered if withdrawal symptoms are present or the patient's urine contains opioids. Naloxone may be administered intravenously or subcutaneously. *If the intravenous route is used*, one fourth of the total dose should be administered and the patient observed for 30 seconds for withdrawal symptoms; if none occurs, the remainder of the dose should be administered and the patient observed for 20 minutes. *If the subcutaneous route is used*, the full dose should be administered and the patient observed for 45 minutes for withdrawal symptoms. If withdrawal symptoms occur, the naloxone challenge should be repeated at 24-hour intervals until absence of opioid dependence is confirmed.

3. Charcoal is generally ineffective in absorbing *small ionic compounds*, like lithium, Mg, arsenic, alcohols (*hemodialysis is better* for these compounds). Charcoal should also not be given for caustic ingestion.

13. In digoxin toxicity atropine is often effective for bradycardias, and lidocaine or dilantin are *preferred* for ventricular irritability. The use of digoxin-specific Fab fragments (Digibind®) is reserved for *severe* intoxication—it binds the digoxin making it incapable of binding at its receptor, the Na+/K+-ATPase.

14. Tricyclic antidepressant overdose is actually one of the most serious types of OD and accounts for 25% of all deaths due to poisoning.

ACID-BASE DISORDERS

2. The patient has a metabolic alkalosis with adequate respiratory compensation as can be appreciated by the similarity of the last 2 digits of the pH to the pCO_2. The first step in understanding a metabolic alkalosis is to check the urine chloride. A urine chloride of less than 10 is referred to as a 'chloride-sensitive' metabolic alkalosis. You might remember this by the fact that the patient responds to, or is 'sensitive' to, the administration of NaCL since the main causes of a urine chloride <10 include GI/renal losses. On the contrary, a urine chloride > 10 is referred to as a 'chloride-resistant', or 'chloride-unresponsive' metabolic alkalosis, and includes a wider variety of etiologies discussed below.

3. Bartter's syndrome, hyperaldosteronism, and Cushing's syndrome are all examples of chloride-resistant metabolic alkalosis (urine CL>10). In Bartter's syndrome, the blood pressure is usually low/normal, but is elevated in hyperaldosteronism, Cushing's syndrome and renal artery stenosis.

4. When the PaO_2 increases with an increase in the FIO_2, there's no shunt, and the key differentials include asthma, interstitial lung disease, and PE. Pneumonia is an example of perfused but unventilated/poorly ventilated alveoli, and there is a shunt. Other examples of shunts include aspiration, edema (CHF), and pulmonary hemorrhage, all intrapulmonary shunts, wherein the PaO_2 does not fully correct with an increase in the FIO_2. Examples of intracardiac shunts (less common than intrapulmonary shunts) would be ASD and VSD.

5-7. The expression "delta-delta" refers to the change in anion gap divided by the change in HCO_3-. It should be calculated whenever you have an increased anion gap metabolic acidosis. Basically, it's done in order to figure out if there's a second underlying disorder, i.e. a mixed disorder. In general, for every ↑ in the AG, there is an equal ↓ in the HCO_3^-, so...

- **If the delta-delta<1**, that means there's A "CONCEALED" (or additional hidden) *NON-ANION GAP METABOLIC ACIDOSIS*. Why? Because < 1 implies that the change in the bicarb was greater than the change in the AG. That means the ↓ in bicarb was more than expected for the anion gap alone.

and...

- **If the delta-delta is > 1**, that means there's a CONCEALED *METABOLIC ALKALOSIS*. The logic is the same.

    - ***For example (!)***, given the upper limit of a normal AG is 12, if the patient's AG = 20, the Δ AG = 8, so we'd expect a Δ HCO_3^- to be the same, or (24-X) = 8, so "X", or the measured HCO_3^- should =16. If it's < 16, the delta-delta will be <1, and there must be a concealed non-anion gap metabolic acidosis. If the measured HCO_3^- >16, the delta-delta >1, so there must be an additional metabolic alkalosis .

8. If the patient's AG = 20, the Δ AG=8, so we'd expect a Δ HCO_3^- to be the same, or (24-X) = 8, so "X", or the measured HCO_3^- should =16. But this patient's measured HCO_3^- >16, making the delta-delta >1, so there must be an additional metabolic alkalosis.

13. Respiratory compensation formulas can be summarized in the following easy Quick-Chart™ table. Use compensation formulas to figure out the expected HCO_3^-. If HCO_3^- is more or less than the expected compensation, **there's *another* primary process going on**!

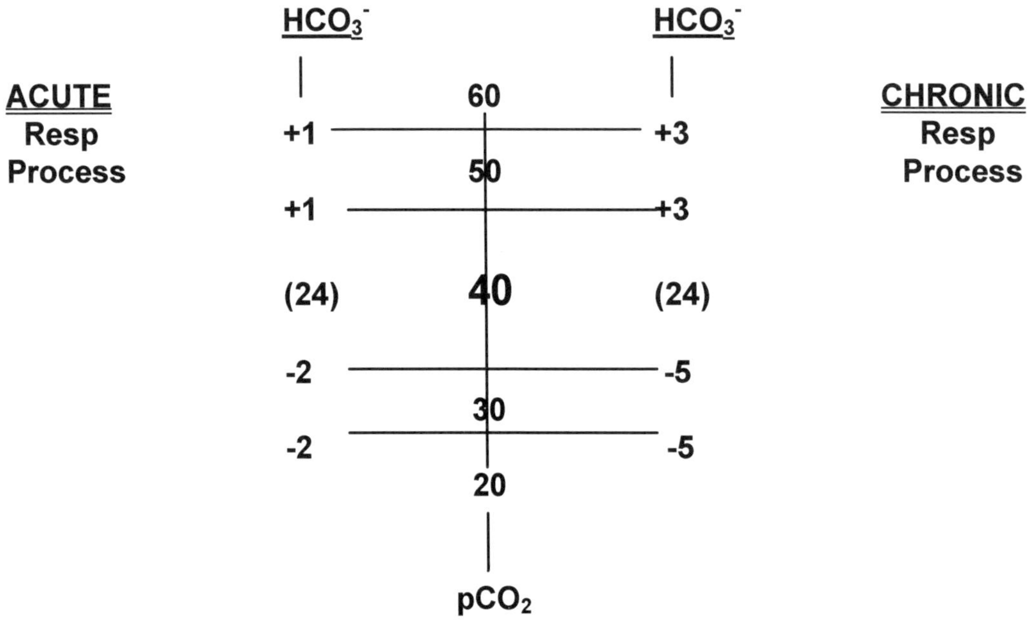

NOTE: *The "+1, +3, -2, and -5" are the amounts that should be added or subtracted from 24 to calculate the true HCO_3^-.* This Quick-Chart ™ works as follows: "for every 10" that the pCO2 is above or below 40, you add or subtract the given amounts (1, 2, 3, or 5) to get your expected HCO3⁻. Then you compare that number to the labs value to unmask any additional primary processes going on.

LET'S TAKE SOME EXAMPLES ..

- If a patient is in ACUTE respiratory distress (refer to the LEFT SIDE of the Quick-Chart™), and her pCO_2 is 20, you see that the bicarb should be 24-2-2more, which=20! If her bicarb is any more or less, there is *another primary* process going on. If her bicarb is 20, then her bicarb is appropriately compensated and the process is straightforward.

- If a patient is in <u>ACUTE</u> respiratory distress and he becomes lethargic, and his pCO_2 is 60, you see that the bicarb should be 24 +1 +1 more, which=26, again if appropriately compensated and assuming no additional contributing process.

- If a patient is in <u>CHRONIC</u> respiratory distress (refer to the <u>RIGHT SIDE</u> of the Quick-Chart™), and his pCO_2 is 30, you see that the bicarb should be 24 - 5, or 19.

- If a patient is in <u>CHRONIC</u> respiratory distress, and his pCO_2 is 50, you see that the bicarb should be 24 +3, or 27.

27. Anemia affects oxygen content only, not oxygen saturation or PaO_2. Carbon monoxide poisoning and abnormal Hgb affinity affect only oxygen saturation and content, not PaO_2. Oxygen content in normal blood can be determined by adding the amount of O_2 dissolved in plasma to the amount bound to hemoglobin, according to the equation: <u>Oxygen content = 1.34 x Hgb x sat + .0031 x PaO2</u> since each gram of hemoglobin is capable of carrying 1.34 mL O_2 when fully saturated, and the amount of O_2 that can be dissolved in plasma is proportional to the PO_2, with 0.0031 mL O_2 dissolved per deciliter of blood per mmHg PO_2. In arterial blood, the amount of O_2 transported dissolved in plasma (approximately 0.3 mL O_2 per deciliter of blood) is trivial compared with the amount bound to hemoglobin (approximately 20 mL O_2 per deciliter of blood).

28. At first glance it appears there is no acid-base disorder and that, beyond the BUN and creatinine, there is no obvious abnormality. However, since you're given the SMA, it's appropriate to check for an anion gap. The AG is approximately 29 which indicates there is a high anion gap metabolic acidosis. Now, whenever you have an anion gap metabolic acidosis you should always calculate the "delta-delta" to determine if there's an additional or 'concealed' metabolic alkalosis *or* non-anion gap metabolic acidosis. The delta-delta is calculated by seeing how much change there is in the bicarbonate relative to the change in AG. In other words, is there more or less bicarb than would be expected. Normally, the change in anion gap should equal the change in bicarb; that is, $\Delta AG/\Delta HCO_3^-$ should be about 1. That's using a normal AG of 12 and a normal bicarb of 24. An easier way to look at it is as a subtraction, instead of a division. In other words, ΔAG minus ΔBG *should* =0. If there's excess HCO_3^-, then there is a *concealed* metabolic alkalosis. If, on the other hand, the AG > BG, then there's a concealed non-anion gap metabolic acidosis. So, when you calculate it out, (normal AG-measured AG)-(normal bicarb-measured bicarb)=(29-12)-(24-24) = +17, <u>*meaning the measured bicarbonate is 17 mEq/L higher than expected for the excess AG, indicating, in addition to the basic anion gap metabolic acidosis, a concealed metabolic alkalosis*</u>! If you'll play through a few of these (and use the subtraction method) you'll see it's actually not as big a deal as you might have thought.

29. Carbon monoxide does not lower the PaO_2.

30. See the explanation to #28 above for the basics on the delta-delta and the bicarbonate gap and it's significance. you can calculate first an AG of 30

    (there's your anion gap metabolic acidosis). *Then* notice that there is an abbreviated, much easier way to calculate the delta-delta: If you work it out, the AG-BG or the "delta-delta" can actually be expressed in much simpler way, and that is: Na-Cl-39, or in this patient: 153-100-39=14 mEq/L, so there is an excess of bicarb (there's your metabolic alkalosis). A normal BG is $\pm$ 6. Therefore, from the electrolytes alone (!) and without the ABG even (!) we can see that there is both an anion gap acidosis and a metabolic alkalosis as well.

31. Natural aging of the lung tissues and subsequent V/Q imbalance causes the PaO_2 to fall with age. However, the alveolar PO_2 stays the same since it is simply a function of barometric pressure, PCO_2, temperature, and fraction of inspired oxygen. Therefore the alveolar-arterial PO_2 difference or "A-a gradient" increases with age. The $PaCO_2$ does not change with age, since it's simply a function of the medullary brainstem, which remains constant.

32. It might even *exacerbate* severe respiratory acidosis by causing a decrease in minute ventilation.

34. See #30 for explanation.

35. When the pO_2 is high, lower the FIO_2. Again, use the Rule of 7's to guide your adjustment in FIO_2: For every 1% decrease in FIO_2, the pO_2 will drop by 7. So, for example, if the pO_2 is 310 on 80% FIO_2, take 310-100 (goal)=210, which is the amount of decrease we will need to make in the pO_2. Dividing 210 by 7, we see we need to lower the FIO_2 by 30. So 80%-30% leaves 50%, which is where we should order the new FIO_2 in order to bring down the pO_2 to 100. If the pO_2 is high and your FIO_2 is already low, then the PEEP can be lowered (usually in increments of 2 with follow-up blood gases). Because of oxygen toxicity, patients with a high pO_2 should have their FIO_2 lowered first, then the PEEP.

36. The FIO_2 remains the same with increasing altitude. Patient's become hypoxemic, and dyspneic because of the decrease in barometric pressure.

38. You need at least two of the three variables in the Henderson-Hasselbach equation to assess the acid-base state of the individual. For purposes of this explanation only (and not to memorize the formula!), the equation goes:

$$pH = 6.1 + \log \frac{HCO_3^-}{PaCO_2 \times .03}$$

39. The pulse oximeter in not equal in accuracy to the co-oximeter, since the co-oximeter uses four wavelengths of light to differentiate Hgb moieties; the pulse ox, on the other hand, uses only two wavelengths, and reads oxyHgb and carboxyHgb together. The end-tidal PCO_2 is usually less than or equal to the $PaCO_2$. In situations of V/Q imbalance, an excess of dead space yields air that has low or no PCO_2 to the end-tidal sample, so that end-tidal PCO_2's are usually lower than $PaCO_2$.

41. As there is an increase in PaO_2 with an increase in the FIO_2, there cannot be a shunt, as is seen with an atrial septal defect (right-to-left shunt).

42. This time, there must be a shunt since there is no real move in the PaO_2, given the ↑ in FIO_2%. All of the answers except c) are included in the potential differential. Narcotic overdose with subsequent hypoventilation is also not possible given this patient's normal $PaCO_2$. In hypoventilation there would be a marked respiratory acidosis.

43. Not only does this patient display a perfectly compensated metabolic alkalosis (pH 7.$\underline{58}$, $PaCO_2$ $\underline{58}$), but she also clearly demonstrates a "contraction alkalosis", with her elevated HCO_3 and depressed chloride. This is not uncommon in cases of volume loss.

44. Lactic acidosis, remember, is the most common cause of a rapid onset, high anion gap metabolic alkalosis. In this firefighter this is happening secondary to the carboxyhemoglobinemia.

STATISTICS

Here's a quick statistics "refresher" to help you answer these questions…

ALWAYS SET UP YOUR 2X2 TABLE THIS WAY:

"GOLD STANDARD" (i.e. the IDEAL test)

	Disease PRESENT	Disease ABSENT
Diagnostic TEST +	**TRUE + "a"**	**False + "b"**
Diagnostic TEST -	**False - "c"**	**TRUE - "d"**

IMPORTANT NOTES:

1. Don't put the headings on the wrong axis
2. **The most important players are "a" and "d"**—Don't forget that!
3. **Sensitivity** goes **down the 1st column**!
4. **Specificity** goes **down the 2nd column!**
5. **Positive Predictive Value (PPV)** goes **across the 1st row!**
6. **Negative Predictive Value (NPV)** goes **across the 2nd row!**

Now That You Know What Each Box Represents (True Positives, True Negatives, Etc), Set It Up Again To Your Advantage ! ☞ 'A' & 'D' ARE THE MOST IMPORTANT! THAT'S WHY THEY'RE IN CAPS & ALWAYS ON TOP!! …

A	**b**	→	**PPV= A/a+b**
c	**D**	→	**NPV= D/c+d**
↓	↓		

Sensitivity=A/a+c

Specificity= D/b+d

PREVALENCE= a+c/a+b+c+d

So, let's look at question #1:

- **You're given a new diagnostic test that gives abnormal results 80% of patients who have the disease but gives normal results in 95% of patients who are truly disease-free. We also tell you that the prevalence of the disease in the population being tested is 10%. You're asked what % of patients who test + actually have the disease (asking Positive Predictive Value).**

WE NOW HAVE EVERYTHING WE NEED:

1. Sensitivity = 80%
2. Specificity = 95%
3. Prevalence = 10%

...which is what we need to set up our 2x2 table and fill in the blanks.

1. Here's the stepwise approach you should always use:

FIRST: Start with the prevalence and arbitrarily assume a population of 100. Well, that means a+b+c+d=100; so 10% of that population is the prevalence.

SECOND: That means a+c =10, since those are the ones who actually have the disease.

THIRD: So, we start picking them off one at a time. If a+c=10, and the sensitivity is 80%, that means "a" must = 8; and therefore "c" must =2. Remember, we're setting this all up so we can calculate the PPV in *percent (!) so don't worry.*

FOURTH: 100 minus 10 (which was a+c, remember) gives us 90, which must =b+d. Now we punch in the specificity, which is 95%, so d/b+d, or d/90=95%. That means "d"= 85.5 (don't worry that's 855 if you arbitrarily chose a population of 1000), so "b" must = 90-85.5 =4.5

FINALLY: So, we now have all the values for "a","b","c", and "d", and we can calculate either PPV or NPV, whatever is asked. Our example asked for **NPV**, so that's d/c+d, or 85.5/90, which is **95%**.

2. This question is solved the exact same way. Just plug in the new sensitivity, specificity, and prevalence, and be sure to use the formula for PPV at the end: PPV=a/a+b. An abbreviated version of the above explanation follows: Assuming a population of 100, knowing the prevalence=25% means that 25%=a+c/100, so a+c=25. Now, since sensitivity=68%=a/a+c and we already know a+c=25, that means a=17. So c must =8 since a+c=25 remember. So we've solved a & c. Next we use the specificity=96%=d/b+d, that is 96%=d/75 since 100-(a+c)=100-25=75. Therefore 96%=d/75 and d must=72. Therefore since we just said the sum of b&d=75, b must =3. So we have a, b, c, and d solved. All we have to do now is plug a & b into the PPV formula since that's what is wanted. **PPV**=17/17+3=17/20= **85%.**

REFERENCES

1. Frontrunners' WEEKEND MARATHON REVIEWS, 1996-2003, Frontrunners Board Review, Inc., New York/California.
2. FRONTRUNNERS' INTERNAL MEDICINE BOARD REVIEW SYLLABUS, Frontrunners Board Review, Inc, Aliso Viejo, CA, © 2003
3. TURBO MNEMONICS: Memory Aids To Commonly Asked Clinical Material You *Gotta* Know For The Boards, 3rd edition, Frontrunners Publishing, Aliso Viejo, CA, © 2003
4. Frontrunners Ultimate Internal Medicine Board Review Course, 1996-2002, New York.
5. NAIL THE BOARDS!, 3rd edition, Frontrunners Publishing, Aliso Viejo, CA, © 2003
6. Harrison's Principles of Internal Medicine 15th edition, McGraw Hill Inc., New York, © 2001 by McGraw Hill Inc.
7. Cecil Essentials of Medicine, 5th edition, Andreoli, T. et al, W. B. Saunders Company, Philadelphia, PA © 2001.
8. ACP Board Review Course, 1996-2003.
9. Medical Knowledge Self Assessment Program VII, VIII, IX, X, XI, and XII, XII update, American College of Physicians, Philadelphia, PA.
10. Heart Disease- A Textbook of Cardiovascular Medicine, edited by Eugene Braunwald, MD, 6th ed, W.B. Saunders Company, © 2001
11. The Sanford Guide to Antimicrobial Therapy 2002, David N. Gilbert, MD, et al, 32nd ed., © 2002.

Quick Order Form

Quick Order Form

YOU SHOULD KNOW WE ALSO OFFER THESE INCREDIBLE RESOURCES !! :

(Put an "X thru the boxes of the products you're interested in)

❒ **WEEKEND MARATHON REVIEWS ™:** ☞ **2003 REVIEWS:**

- **SAT/SUN REVIEWS ! !** ☞ **18 hours:** Key Slides & What You'll Need To Know: **APRIL / AUGUST / OCT 2003**. Call for dates & locations! ☞ Tuition $575

❒ **NAIL THE BOARDS! The *ULTIMATE* Internal Medicine Board Review for Board Exams, © 2003**; *Order for your students or friends!* ☞ $89.95

❒ **INTERNAL MEDICINE Q&A REVIEW: © 2003,** contains > **1200 Q&A** to Prepare You for the Boards! ☞ $149.00

❒ **TURBO MNEMONICS FOR THE BOARDS: MEMORY AIDS TO COMMONLY ASKED CLINICAL MATERIAL ON THE BOARDS**
© **2003**, > ***400 of the BEST Anagrams, Mnemonics, & Time-saving Tricks*** *to BOOST your clinical & boards PERFORMANCE!* ☞ $39.95
+ S&H*: $8.00

4 EASY ORDER OPTIONS: **TOTAL** ☞ ☐

1. ***Fax*** orders: **949-203-6178. FAX THIS FORM.**
2. ***E-mail*** **(or info):** **FRONTRUNNERS@hotmail.com** (safe & reliable)
3. ***Tel.***: **CALL 866-MDBOARDs**. V/MC/AMEX/Discover/Diners
4. ***By mail***: FRONTRUNNERS PUBLISHING/FBRI
   23511 Aliso Creek Rd. Suite 93
   Aliso Viejo, CA 92656

SHIPPING ADDRESS: (Sales tax of 7.75% will be added for all orders shipped within California)
(* Add $8.00 S&H on all orders)

Name: ______________________________

Address: ______________________________

City State Zip: ______________________________

Telephone: ______________________________(for backup *only*)

FAX / EMAIL: ______________________________

(We can ALSO FAX your receipt /confirmation of registration to you within 24h)

PAYMENT OPTIONS: ❒ Money Order ❒ Circle CC: **V/MC/AMEX/Discover/Diners**

Card number: ______________________________

Name on card: ____________________ Exp. Date __________